S. Hrg. 114–112

DEMANDING RESULTS TO END NATIVE YOUTH SUICIDES

HEARING

BEFORE THE

COMMITTEE ON INDIAN AFFAIRS UNITED STATES SENATE

ONE HUNDRED FOURTEENTH CONGRESS

FIRST SESSION

JUNE 24, 2015

Printed for the use of the Committee on Indian Affairs

U.S. GOVERNMENT PUBLISHING OFFICE

97–503 PDF   WASHINGTON : 2015

For sale by the Superintendent of Documents, U.S. Government Publishing Office
Internet: bookstore.gpo.gov   Phone: toll free (866) 512–1800; DC area (202) 512–1800
Fax: (202) 512–2104   Mail: Stop IDCC, Washington, DC 20402–0001

CONTENTS

DEMANDING RESULTS TO END NATIVE YOUTH SUICIDES

WEDNESDAY, JUNE 24, 2015

U.S. SENATE,
COMMITTEE ON INDIAN AFFAIRS,
Washington, DC.

The Committee met, pursuant to notice, at 2:30 p.m. in room 628, Dirksen Senate Office Building, Hon. John Barrasso, Chairman of the Committee, presiding.

OPENING STATEMENT OF HON. JOHN BARRASSO, U.S. SENATOR FROM WYOMING

The CHAIRMAN. Good afternoon. I call this hearing to order.

Today, the Committee will hold an oversight hearing entitled Demanding Results to End Native Youth Suicides.

Over the past ten years, this Committee has held six formal hearings to address the issue of youth suicide. We return to this panel issue once again today because youth suicide continues to plague too many Indian communities.

In 2011, the Substance Abuse and Mental Health Services Administration identified youth suicide as the second leading cause of death for Indian youth between 15 and 24 years of age. The U.S. Centers for Disease Control reported Native youth suicide to be two and a half times the national average in 2012.

Some communities are dealing with daily suicide attempts and suicide clusters. Over the last six months, the Pine Ridge Indian Reservation in South Dakota has suffered at least 11 suicides and at least 379 suicide attempts have been reported.

I was troubled to learn from the testimony submitted by President Steele that a youth pastor at the Pine Ridge Reservation received word that a group of children had planned a group suicide. The pastor sped to the place it was planned and found many ropes hanging from the trees.

Thankfully, the pastor arrived before any of the children attempted to hang themselves. He was able to counsel them on the spot, undoubtedly saving their lives in the process.

This is just one reservation. Many communities across Indian Country are facing similar tragedies or attempted tragedies. Our hearts go out to the families and communities for their great losses.

I will not stand idly by, nor will this Committee. There must be a better way of supporting the young people, parents, teachers and community leaders that are fighting against suicide. We all share

(1)

the goal of ending youth suicides in Indian Country. Achieving this goal requires a comprehensive and evidence-based plan that is proactive instead of reactive.

I am very concerned that the Administration's plan and actions so far have been insufficient. The Department of Health and Human Services is responsible for the delivery of health services to American Indians and Alaska Natives. Its duty is to uphold the Federal obligation to promote healthy Indian communities and honor tribal governance, but it has failed to do so.

I talked directly with Secretary Burwell last week. She shares our concern. Native youth suicide is too significant a threat for this Committee to accept anything less than measurable results.

I am very troubled that Federal agencies with responsibilities to American Indians and Alaska Natives do not seem to be learning from the tribes like the White Mountain Apache Tribe and the Menominee Indian Tribe of Wisconsin which have actually reduced the number of suicides in their communities.

We will not turn away from this issue until it is resolved. The time for finger pointing, lack of coordination and excuses is over. This Committee will do whatever it takes legislatively and in its oversight capacity to support results.

Today, we will hear testimony from tribal leaders, a subject matter expert and the Administration.

Speaking of the Administration, a lot of time and energy has been spent in preparing for this hearing today. It is unacceptable that the Committee only received the Administration's testimony late yesterday afternoon.

I want to welcome our panel and look forward to hearing their perspectives.

Before we hear from the panel, I want to thank Vice Chairman Tester for his attention to the issue and invite him to make an opening statement.

STATEMENT OF HON. JON TESTER, U.S. SENATOR FROM MONTANA

Senator TESTER. Thank you, Mr. Chairman. Thank you for holding this hearing today.

I would join you in your resolve to get this issue on youth suicide and suicide in Indian Country settled. I appreciate anything we can do to work together to truly make some inroads.

This is a bad issue. My friend and former Chairman of this Committee, Senator Dorgan, who retired in 2011, put a good amount of time into solving this issue. It still is an epidemic among tribal nations across this country.

As we have heard at our Committee hearings over and over again, children in Indian Country face some dreadful realities. Late last year, the Department of Justice releases a report called Ending Violence So Children Can Survive. Included in that report was a finding that Native children experience PTSD at the same rate as veterans from the wars in Iraq and Afghanistan. We have some problems. To say that this is troubling does not even begin to characterize the situation.

Many of our Native children face hopelessness each and every day. They wake up to overcrowded homes with up to 10 or 15 people living in a two or three bedroom house. Many lack access to fresh, healthy food or breakfast because they live in food deserts.

These youths get on school buses sometimes traveling for an hour or more to get to schools that are often run down and lack available staff to teach and nurture them. We have had hearings on this also.

These are just some of the challenges Native children face every day. This is all before lunch.

There is no single, simple solution. We need to work together to improve everything from nutrition to housing to health care to public safety. I am grateful to see this Administration has formed a Council on Native American Affairs. This is a more holistic approach to addressing the needs of Native communities. It will help remove the bureaucratic red tape that has been in place for far too long.

We cannot continue to air drop in resources erratically when suicides spike in Indian communities and turn around and abandon those communities when patchwork funding runs out. We need stability, consistency in mental health programs and a community effort to remove the stigma associated with mental health and mental health treatment.

In my home State of Montana, sadly, this issue is not new. On the Fort Peck Indian Reservation, the tribe was faced with a wave of suicides in recent years and has since developed a suicide prevention plan.

That plan includes significant steps to address risk factors, implement prevention efforts and develop a crisis response plan. Interestingly, many tribes are finding that increased access and exposure to culture and language resources promotes a positive self image and improves mental health for Native youth. Fort Peck's plan also focuses on ways to increase community knowledge on how to assess risk in order to refer individuals for treatment and increased access to appropriate preventative care.

Tribes know what they need. Many are in the position to implement programs to support these efforts. What they lack is a sustainable funding source. These efforts are at the heart of the trust responsibility our government holds with tribal nations.

Now the Federal Government needs to step up and do what we need to do to support tribes in their efforts to stop this awful cycle. Unfortunately, this year it seems like we can provide more money for defense budgets but we cannot put more money into saving lives of Native youth. This is unacceptable by anybody's standard.

I look forward to the testimony of the witnesses today to hear what we can do to work together to help end this youth suicide epidemic.

I want to thank the panelists for being here today. I know some of you have been through some very difficult times recently. You all know this issue inside and out. I look forward to your testimony.

Thank you, Mr. Chairman.

The CHAIRMAN. Thank you, Senator Tester.

Would any other members like to make a statement? Senator Heitkamp.

STATEMENT OF HON. HEIDI HEITKAMP,
U.S. SENATOR FROM NORTH DAKOTA

Senator HEITKAMP. Thank you, Mr. Chairman and Vice Chairman Tester.

Once again, here we are, wringing our hands and telling deplorable and horrible stories of situations that should shock the Nation's conscience but somehow do not ever seem to filter out of this hearing room.

This is not a new issue. During my time serving as North Dakota's Attorney General, we had a high rate of suicide in Indian Country but it has become almost epidemic. We cannot simply say "we share your concern." It is not enough any longer for the Federal Government to say we share the concerns of all the tribal entities and all the tribal families and all the tribal parents who are losing the next generation of their children. We must take action. The unfortunate thing is frequently that action we must take involves resources, involves community coming together, having enough resources, and having a great plan.

Mr. Chairman, I welcome all of the wonderful witnesses we have today here to talk about an extraordinarily difficult subject, I am very interested in hearing what successful practices and models Dr. Teresa D. LaFromboise has to share, because we have to find a solution. We have to find best practices and then we have to fund those best practices.

I want to personally thank Dr. LaFromboise for being here. She is of Miami tribal decent and is the proud mother of her daughter, Cecily, who is an enrolled member at the Turtle Mountain Band of Chippewa located in North Dakota. I think her expertise and her commitment will be revealed in her testimony. I am particularly anxious to hear what steps we need to take, when we need to take them and how we change this dynamic. What we have done in the past, taking a look at the rapid increases that we have seen, what we have done in the past clearly has not worked.

Thank you, Mr. Chairman. You continue to have my participation and my commitment to work with you and with the Vice Chairman on a path forward.

The CHAIRMAN. Thank you, Senator Heitkamp.

Senator Udall?

STATEMENT OF HON. TOM UDALL,
U.S. SENATOR FROM NEW MEXICO

Senator UDALL. Thank you very much, Chairman Barrasso and Vice Chairman Tester. I really appreciate your pulling this hearing together on this incredibly important subject.

The loss of one child's life is debilitating for families and I think for the entire community. In my home State of New Mexico, we have lost far too many young people in our Native communities.

As Senator Heitkamp discussed, when I was Attorney General in New Mexico and then a Congressman before I came to the Senate, the numbers were way, way too high. Just to throw one at you, the New Mexico Department of Health estimates that at least 201 Native American youth have died of suicide between 1999 and 2013.

There has been evidence of suicide clusters, a series of two or three suicides in the community over the course of the year or less occurring on the Mescalero Apache Indian Reservation and also the Eastern Navajo Nation. It is likely that the statistics are significantly under-counting these tragedies.

There are also high concentrations of risk factors in New Mexico's Native communities. Last year, in a survey of 1,300 Native Americans from seven different tribal communities in the State, the University of New Mexico researchers found that 29 percent had been exposed to four or more traumatic experiences as children such as alcohol and drug abuse, physical violence at home, neglect, abuse, separated or divorced parents or a close family member in prison.

It is critical that we listen to our Native youth and remove the stigma from talking about suicide and trauma. We must create and sustain opportunities for them to learn the value of their cultures and identities.

We need to make sure they are connected to adequate mental health services. We must show them that their lives matter.

I want to thank the witnesses for being here today and for all the hard work they have done in their communities and the crises that are occurring around the country. We must do better.

Thank you very much, Mr. Chairman.

The CHAIRMAN. Thank you.

We will now hear from our witnesses. We have with us today the Honorable Robert G. McSwain, Acting Director, Indian Health Service, U.S. Department of Health and Human Services, Rockville, Maryland. We have the Honorable Collins "C.J." Clifford, Tribal Council Member, Oglala Sioux Tribe of Pine Ridge, South Dakota. Councilman Clifford is filling in for President Steele. We also have the Honorable Darrell G. Seki, Sr., Chairman, Red Lake Band of Chippewa Indians, Red Lake, Minnesota, and Teresa D. LaFromboise, P.h.D, Professor, Developmental and Psychological Sciences, Graduate School of Education, Stanford University, Stanford, California.

I thank you all for being here. I want to remind our witnesses that your full written testimony will be made a part of the official hearing record. Please keep your statements to five minutes so that we may have time for questions. I look forward to hearing your testimony, beginning with Mr. McSwain.

STATEMENT OF HON. ROBERT G. MCSWAIN, ACTING DIRECTOR, INDIAN HEALTH SERVICE, U.S. DEPARTMENT OF HEALTH AND HUMAN SERVICES

Mr. MCSWAIN. Mr. Chairman, Vice Chairman and members of the Committee, good afternoon.

I am Robert McSwain, current Acting Director of the Indian Health Service. I appreciate the opportunity to testify on demanding results to end Native youth suicide.

I agree, number one, this is a very serious issue. I have been talking with Councilman Clifford as we prepared for the hearing about how things are going. I have not had a chance to talk with President Steele this week but I try to call him every week.

I would just highlight some of the key programs, initiatives and investments that we are doing to end youth suicide. I look forward to continuing to work with the Committee, as you have offered.

As you know, Indian Health Service, of any group plays a rather unique role. We are providing health care and we are sitting on the reservation. I have some comments about how we can make that even better.

The mission of the Indian Health Service is to raise the physical, mental, social and spiritual health of American Indians and Alaska Natives to the highest possible level. That is our mission and has been for the last 20 years. I just want to restate that.

You mentioned some statistics and I am not going to go through all of those. You are probably well aware of it. I will say we have published a new Trends in Indian Health dated 2014. It is on our website. We have recited all of those particular notations you have made in the case of suicide which is the sixth leading cause of death overall for males residing in IHS service areas. I think that is a real issue.

I want to say that when tribal leaders often request help from us in many different forms, either funding or during a cluster, we generally will respond immediately whether it is funding to help locally or if they have asked for deployments. We have done that.

In fact, in the deployments to Pine Ridge, we were able to convene a deployment within a week to go to Pine Ridge. We had three cycles of folks up there. As you mentioned, Mr. Chairman, it was only temporary as we move ahead. We need to do something more substantial.

The most important part I can say today is the fact that this year we will launch the Zero Suicide Initiative. The most important part of this concept is as patients go through our clinics, we have to have our folks trained to identify where the at-risk youth are coming to us, know when to see it and when to be able to have that conversation. We are a health system and they come to us for a lot of reasons. We ought to be able to monitor the youth better.

I would just enumerate the other parts because you have it in my statement. We have a Meth Suicide Prevention Initiative. That has been going on for six years. We will get the results this year. That is community-based.

There are 130 programs across the Nation. Domestic violence is another initiative that is community-based. These are important pieces we are putting in place. They had 65 projects and certainly the DVPI expands outreach.

Prioritizing health care for youth is one I am very excited about. We are going to jump ahead. It is in the President's budget for 2016 but we are going to go ahead and open a Pathways program and begin to hire Native youth to work in our facilities and service units to get them doing something different and perhaps expose them to health care and forming youth steering committees so they can get together and begin to share.

There was a comment about lack of integration. We are working closely with the Substance Abuse and Mental Health Administration. A good example of our response to Pine Ridge is that we are working on our health system to improve it and make it more responsive and SAMHSA is providing support to help the community work their piece of it. This is a two-part process.

The other part is behavioral health. We have turned on Tele-Behavioral Health to Pine Ridge, for example, and to the outlying clinics so that we can provide access to care locally in some of those health centers.

I will also mention the biggest challenge we will have in rural America is recruit and retention of health care providers. We ran up against this at Pine Ridge and immediately we had a problem with housing. We did a little work-around. I won't go into how we did the work-around, but we were able to provide temporary housing for staff that desperately needed to be on-site.

We will do more in this area. I think there will be questions about health care professionals that we need in the area, certainly behavioral health folks. We are working on that very diligently.

I think we have some pieces that we are putting together that will integrate all of the pieces. We have all these programs. We just want to have one place where they are all working together and not working in silos or separately.

With that, I will close my oral remarks.

[The prepared statement of Mr. McSwain follows:]

PREPARED STATEMENT OF HON. ROBERT G. MCSWAIN, ACTING DIRECTOR, INDIAN HEALTH SERVICE, U.S. DEPARTMENT OF HEALTH AND HUMAN SERVICES

Chairman and Members of the Committee:

Good afternoon, I am Robert G. McSwain, Acting Director of the Indian Health Service (IHS). Today, I appreciate the opportunity to testify on "Demanding Results to End Native Youth Suicide."

Thank you for the invitation to talk about this very serious issue of Native youth suicide. It is with a heavy heart that we discuss an issue that continues to plague American Indian and Alaska Native (AI/AN) communities. Most recently, the Oglala Sioux Tribe has faced the same tragedy of a suicide cluster that too many other AI/AN communities have experienced. Our thoughts go out to the Oglala Sioux Tribe and the families and friends who are grieving the loss of their young people. Today, I will highlight our key programs, initiatives, and investments to end Native youth suicide and we look forward to continuing to work with the Committee to address this devastating problem.

As you know, the Indian Health Service (IHS) plays a unique role in the Department of Health and Human Services because it is a health care system that was established to meet the federal trust responsibility to provide health care to American Indians and Alaska Natives. The IHS provides high-quality, comprehensive primary care and public health services through a system of IHS, Tribal, and Urban operated facilities and programs based on treaties, judicial determinations, and Acts of Congress. The IHS has the responsibility for the delivery of health services to an estimated 2.2 million American Indians and Alaska Natives who belong to 566 Federally-recognized Tribes. The mission of the agency is to raise the physical, mental, social, and spiritual health of American Indians and Alaska Natives to the highest level. The agency goal is to assure that comprehensive, culturally appropriate personal and public health services are available and accessible to the AI/AN population. Our duty is to uphold the Federal Government's obligation to promote healthy AI/AN people, communities, and cultures and to honor and protect the inherent sovereign rights of Tribes.

Two major pieces of legislation are at the core of the Federal Government's responsibility for meeting the health needs of American Indians and Alaska Natives: The Snyder Act of 1921, 25 U.S.C § 13, and the Indian Health Care Improvement Act (IHCIA), 25 U.S.C. §§ 1601–1683. The Snyder Act authorized appropriations for "the relief of distress and conservation of health" of American Indians and Alaska Natives. The IHCIA was enacted "to implement the Federal responsibility for the care and education of the Indian people by improving the services and facilities of Federal Indian health programs and encouraging maximum participation of Indians in such programs." Like the Snyder Act, the IHCIA provides the authority for the provision of programs, services, functions, and activities to address the health needs of American Indians and Alaska Natives. The IHCIA also includes authorities for the recruitment and retention of health professionals serving Indian communities, health services for people, and the construction, replacement, and repair of healthcare facilities.

Introduction

We share your deep concern about the tragedy of suicide among Native youth. Suicide is a complicated public health challenge with many contributing factors in AI/AN communities. Although suicide contagion is not unique to AI/AN populations, too frequently, AI/AN communities experience suicide that takes on a particularly worrying and seemingly contagious form, often referred to as suicide clusters. In these communities, the suicidal act becomes a regular and transmittable form of expression of the despair and hopelessness experienced by some Native youth. While most vividly and painfully expressed in close knit AI/AN communities, suicide and suicidal behavior and their consequences send shockwaves through the community. We at IHS—and at HHS more broadly—try to prevent these suicide clusters from beginning and to halt them once they begin occurring.

However, all too many AI/AN communities are affected by high rates of suicide. The recently published IHS "*Trends in Indian Health, 2014*" reports:

- The age adjusted suicide rate (18.5 per 100,000 population) for the three year period (2007–2009) in the IHS service areas was 1.6 times that of the U.S. all races rate (11.6) for 2008.
- Suicide is the second leading cause of death (behind unintentional injuries) for Indian youth ages 15–24 residing in IHS service areas and the suicide death rate for this cohort is four times higher than the national average.
- Suicide is the sixth leading cause of death overall for males residing in IHS service areas and ranks ahead of homicide.
- AI/AN young people ages 15–34 make up 64 percent of all suicides in Indian country.

Responding to Suicide Crises

Tribal leaders will often request IHS to provide additional support and funding to help prevent any further suicides during a cluster. Since no two suicide clusters are the same, the IHS response is tailored to the needs of the community in crisis. In general, our Area Office typically takes the first steps to organize and implement a response to a suicide crisis. In particular, the IHS Area Office reaches out to tribal leadership to ensure IHS and key Federal partners, such as the Substance Abuse and Mental Health Services Administration (SAMHSA), are aware of the Tribe's level of need and the specific requests for a response. We take steps to work hand-in-hand with the tribe, in organizing our response. IHS and SAMHSA coordinate to ensure Federal resources are readily available.

SAMHSA's resources may include existing grants awarded to the tribe under the new Tribal Behavioral Health Grant (TBHG) program that is focused on preventing suicidal behavior and substance abuse and promoting mental health in AI/AN youth or the Garrett Lee Smith State/Tribal Youth Suicide Prevention program that supports youth suicide prevention and early intervention strategies and collaborations among youth-serving institutions and systems (i.e., schools, juvenile justice, foster care, substance abuse, mental health, and other child and youth supporting organizations). Other SAMHSA resources include specialized technical assistance centers such as the Suicide Prevention Resource Center, National Native Children's Trauma Center, and National AI/AN Addiction Technology Transfer Center.

If the Tribe requests a deployment of healthcare providers, IHS takes the lead with the Division of Commissioned Corps Personnel and Readiness (DCCPR) to assess and plan for the deployment. A deployment team can be on the ground in a matter of days. These short term deployment teams are intended to deal with the immediate crisis until mid- and long-term solutions can be set in place.

Zero Suicide

In 2015, IHS will launch the Zero Suicide Initiative, a key concept of the 2012 National Strategy for Suicide Prevention. In our current system, suicide care has traditionally been provided by individual local champions and clinical providers. IHS is moving toward a more programmatic system-wide approach by implementing Zero Suicide. IHS' commitment to create a leadership-driven, safety-oriented culture committed to reducing suicide among people under our care will drive the improved patient outcomes we need to see as a result of a collective Agency effort. Moving forward, IHS is making the commitment to set big goals and improve our approach to inform system changes to provide better care for AI/AN individuals at risk for suicide.

Zero Suicide represents a bold goal for IHS. It is the foundational belief that suicide deaths for individuals under our care within our health and behavioral health systems are preventable. IHS is committed to creating a leadership-driven, safety-oriented culture focused on reducing suicide. The approach represents a commitment from IHS to set in place an organizational structure where suicidal individuals and individuals at-risk will receive coordinated care from a competent workforce. The fundamentals of Zero Suicide implementation include: leadership's commitment to reduce suicide deaths; training a competent, confident, caring workforce; identifying and assessing patients for suicide risk; engaging patients at risk for suicide in a care plan; treating suicidal thoughts and behaviors directly; following patients through every transition in care; and applying data-driven quality improvement. To accomplish our commitment, IHS has begun a virtual training series through the Tele-Behavioral Health Center of Excellence (TBHCE). IHS is also partnering with SAMHSA and the Suicide Prevention Resource Center to bring a tailored Zero Suicide Training Academy for IHS and Tribal healthcare facilities in 2015. In addition, as discussed below, the Fiscal Year (FY) 2016 Budget requests an additional $25 million to hire additional behavioral health providers through the Methamphetamine and Suicide Prevention Initiative (MSPI).

Methamphetamine and Suicide Prevention Initiative

The MSPI is an IHS nationally-coordinated demonstration project, focusing on providing much-needed methamphetamine and suicide prevention and intervention resources for AI/AN communities. It is a key resource for IHS as we work to prevent youth suicides. It promotes the use and development of evidence-based and practice-based models that represent culturally-appropriate prevention and treatment approaches from a community-driven context.

The MSPI supports 130 programs across the country. The goals of the MSPI are to:

• Prevent, reduce, or delay the use and/or spread of methamphetamine use;
• Build on the foundation of prior methamphetamine and suicide prevention and treatment efforts, in order to support the IHS, Tribes, and Urban Indian health organizations in developing and implementing culturally appropriate methamphetamine and suicide prevention and early intervention strategies;
• Increase access to methamphetamine and suicide prevention services;
• Improve services for behavioral health issues associated with methamphetamine use and suicide prevention;
• Promote the development of new and promising services that are culturally and community relevant; and
• Demonstrate efficacy and impact.

MSPI projects provide multiple services related to suicide and methamphetamine use. The most common focus of funded projects is suicide prevention (94 percent), methamphetamine prevention (69 percent), and suicide treatment and intervention (55 percent). The MSPI projects are in the sixth and final year of the demonstration program. From 2009–2014, the MSPI resulted in over 9,400 individuals entering treatment for methamphetamine use; more than 12,000 encounters via tele-health for substance abuse and mental health disorders; over 13,150 professionals and community members trained in suicide crisis response; and more than 528,000 encounters with youth provided as part of evidence-based and practice-based prevention activities.

MSPI projects offer a multitude of evidence-based practices and treatments. The most common types of evidence-based practices utilized among MSPI programs to prevent suicide are Question, Persuade, Refer (QPR); Applied Suicide Intervention Skills Training (ASIST); Safe Tell, Ask, Listen, Keepsafe (safeTALK); Mental Health First Aid; and Gathering of Native Americans. Evidence-based treatments to prevent suicide re-attempts utilized among MSPI programs include Motivational Interviewing, Cognitive Behavior Therapy (CBT), and Dialectical Behavior Therapy, to name a few. For instance, the White Earth MSPI project, called Native Alive, stations mental health professionals at reservations schools and maintains a support hotline staffed by health professionals trained in ASIST.

MSPI projects often incorporate cultural elements into their programs and activities such as by teaching traditional beliefs, smudging, ceremonies, or sweat lodges in collaboration with traditional healers. The Absentee Shawnee MSPI project, Following in Our Footsteps, utilizes cultural activities such as Native American storytelling, arts and crafts, dancing, sweat lodge ceremonies, and positive youth activities to promote healthy life choices and positive decision-making skills.

Building on the associations between social connections and lower suicide risk, MSPI projects enlist partners to build community-based suicide prevention. Partnerships with local schools are key in the MSPI for school-based interventions to develop skills to protect against suicidal thoughts and behaviors, raise awareness, encourage help-seeking, and teach positive life and coping skills. Examples of such activities at work in MSPI communities include American Indian Life Skills, Native Hope, and Project Venture. Youth may not want or may not always be able to ask appropriate adults for help and may reach out to their peers for assistance. MSPI projects offer training to youth to build their intervention skills for such situations. The MSPI funds allow projects to expand community-based mental health care into youth-based settings, increasing access to care for mental health and substance use disorders for our Native youth. The funding for MSPI funding is not enough to go to every Tribe. Therefore, IHS awards the funds on a competitive basis. In FY 2015, IHS will open a new funding announcement for a project period to run from September 30, 2015 to September 29, 2020, contingent on appropriations.

Domestic Violence Prevention Initiative

Since the Institutes of Medicine (2002) report [1] on suicide research, there has been much learned about the role of child abuse in later suicide risk. According to the Center on the Developing Child at Harvard University, a toxic stress response can occur when a child experiences strong, frequent, and/or prolonged adversity, such as physical or emotional abuse, chronic neglect, caregiver substance use and mental health disorders, exposure to violence, and/or the accumulated burdens of family economic hardship. These adverse childhood experiences can disrupt the development of brain architecture and other organ systems, and increase the risk for stress-related disease and cognitive impairment, well into the adult years.

IHS' primary response to children exposed to violence is through the Domestic Violence Prevention Initiative (DVPI). The IHS began the DVPI in 2010 with the purpose of better addressing domestic violence (DV) and sexual assault (SA), including the pediatric and adolescent population, within AI/AN communities. The program has awarded funding to a total of 65 projects that include IHS/Tribal/Urban operated programs. This initiative promotes the development of evidence-based and practice-based models that represent culturally appropriate prevention and treatment approaches to DV and SA from a community-driven context. Types of evidence-based treatment practices provided by DVPI projects include CBT, Trauma Focused CBT, Beyond Trauma: Traumatic Incident Reduction, and Strengthening Families, a program to improve parenting and family relationships. Practice-based practices utilized by DVPI projects include elders teaching traditions, talking circles, or smudging ceremonies. For instance, Santa Clara Pueblo provides more community education activities; in-school services for young witnesses of family violence; violence prevention education in schools; and counseling for young victims of DV.

The DVPI expands outreach and increases awareness by funding projects that provide victim advocacy, intervention, case coordination, policy development, community response teams, and community and school education programs. The funding is also used for the purchase of forensic equipment, medical personnel training, and the coordination of Sexual Assault Examiner (SAE) and Sexual Assault Response Team activities. From 2010–2014, the DVPI resulted in over 50,500 direct service encounters including crisis intervention, victim advocacy, case management, and counseling services. More than 38,000 referrals were made for domestic violence services, culturally-based services, and clinical behavioral health services. In addition, a total of 600 forensic evidence collection kits from eight SAE programs were submitted to Federal, state, and tribal law enforcement. In the last year, DVPI projects referred over 2,000 children and youth to behavioral health, cultural services, DV or SA services, shelter services, specialized medical care, or to victim advocates.

Prioritizing Behavioral Health Services for Native Youth

The Administration's 2016 Budget proposes key investments to launch Generation Indigenous (Gen-I), an initiative addressing barriers to success for Native American youth. This integrative, comprehensive, and culturally appropriate approach across the Federal Government will help improve lives and opportunities for Native American youth. The HHS Budget Request includes a new Tribal Behavioral Health Initiative for Native Youth with a total of $50 million in funding for IHS and the SAMHSA. Within IHS, the request includes $25 million to expand the successful MSPI to increase the number of child and adolescent behavioral health professionals who will provide direct services and implement youth-based programming at IHS, tribal, and urban Indian health programs, school-based health centers, or youth-based programs. SAMHSA will expand the Tribal Behavioral Health Grant program to support mental health promotion and substance use prevention activities for high-risk Native youth and their families, enhance early detection of mental and substance use disorders among Native youth, and increase referral to treatment.

---

[1] See: *http://www.iom.edu/Reports/2002/Reducing-Suicide-A-National-Imperative.aspx*

These activities will both fill gaps in services and fulfill requests from tribal leaders to support Native youth.

IHS' Gen-I activities include youth engagement through the development of youth steering committees at the local level to inform IHS on planning, implementation, and evaluation of its youth health programs and services. The information from the local youth steering committees will feed into regional and national recommendations to operationalize the input received from Native youth. Secondly, IHS will provide opportunities through its Pathways Internship Program. Pathways is a stream-lined program designed to attract students enrolled in a wide variety of educational institutions (high school, home-school programs, vocational and technical, under-graduate and graduate) with paid opportunities to work in agencies and explore Federal careers while still in school. This program exposes students to jobs in the Federal civil service by providing meaningful "developmental work" at the beginning of their career, before their "career paths" are fully established. The flexible nature of the program is to accommodate the need to hire students to complete temporary work or projects, perform labor intensive tasks not requiring subject matter exper-tise, or to work traditional "summer jobs." The program provides agencies with the opportunity to hire interns who successfully complete the program and academic re-quirements into any competitive service position for which the Intern is qualified. The IHS Gen-I Pathways Internship Program offers Native youth an opportunity to apply for paid summer positions at IHS Service Units in their local community. The initiative kicked off in May 2015, and we have posted job advertisements at all the IHS Areas and have over 80 summer internship positions allocated IHS-wide.

IHS will also provide more funding opportunities geared toward Native youth for early intervention and positive youth development through its three largest initia-tives. In the Special Diabetes Program for Indians, grantees will have the option to elect to use FY 2016 funding to implement the Family Spirit Program, an early intervention home visiting program. Family Spirit is an evidence-based and cul-turally tailored in-home parent training and support program. Parents gain knowl-edge and skills to achieve optimum development for their preschool aged children across the domains of physical, cognitive, social-emotional, language learning, and self-help. The program is currently the largest, most rigorous, and only evidence-based home visiting program ever designed specifically for American Indian fami-lies. Family Spirit now has randomized controlled trial evidence demonstrating that it reduces risk factors associated with a number of adverse outcomes, including obe-sity and substance use.

The MSPI program will also provide FY 2015 funding for local programs to sup-port their Gen-I activities through evidence-based and practice-based programming. Examples of such activities include implementation of American Indian Life Skills, Model Adolescent Suicide Prevention Program, Project Venture, Native HOPE (Helping Our People Endure), ASIST (Applied Suicide Intervention Skills Training), and cultural activities like Native American storytelling, traditional teachings, cere-monies, and other local relevant practices.

Behavioral Health Integration with Primary Care

The current system of services for treating mental health problems of American Indians and Alaska Natives is a complex and often fragmented system of tribal, Federal, state, local, and community-based services. The availability and adequacy of mental health programs for American Indians and Alaska Natives varies consid-erably across communities. The future of AI/AN health depends largely upon how effectively behavioral health is addressed by individuals, families, and communities and how well it is integrated into community health systems. We know that success-ful and sustained behavioral change will require cultural reconnection, community participation, increased resources, leadership capacity, and the ability of systems to be responsive to emerging issues and changing needs. In 2014, IHS began a small pilot project of six sites, the Behavioral Health Integration Initiative (BH2I). The goal of the funding was for sites to develop rapid cycle improvements of behavioral health integration with primary care using the Improving Patient Care (IPC) model. BH2I will continue into FY 2016. IHS will host a National Behavioral Health Inte-gration with Primary Care Conference in Phoenix, Arizona to disseminate integra-tion best practices and lessons learned from BH2I.

The IPC Program is an outpatient primary care quality improvement program de-signed to assist IHS/Tribal/Urban Indian clinics with improving their care delivery and achieving Patient Centered Medical Home (PCMH) recognition. The PCMH is a model of care that aims to transform the delivery of comprehensive primary care to children, adolescents, and adults. The PCMH is best described as a model that is patient-centered, comprehensive, team-based, coordinated, accessible, and focused on quality and safety. The medical home is focused on the needs of patients, and when appropriate, their families and caregivers. A significant element of the PCMH is integration of behavioral health services into primary care patient visits. This can include screening for behavioral health conditions, addressing beliefs about diseases and treatments, identifying disorders and initiating treatment, and collaboration with behavioral health professionals as part of the integrated primary care team.

Training and Tele-Behavioral Health Services

IHS recognizes the need to support access to services and to create a broader range of services linked into a larger network of support and care. IHS piloted the use of tele-behavioral health to increase access to specialty behavioral health services in the MSPI demonstration pilot phase. MSPI projects provided over 6,000 tele-behavioral health encounters in the fifth year alone.

The TBHCE was developed in 2009 to promote and develop tele-behavioral health services. Working in partnership with the University of New Mexico, the TBHCE provides services in a number of settings including school clinics, youth residential treatment centers, and health centers. The TBHCE has leveraged their ability to use federal service providers and provides technical and program support nationally for programs attempting to implement tele-health services. IHS programs are increasingly adopting and using these technologies with more than 8,000 encounters provided via tele-behavioral health in FY 2014.

IHS benefits from the use of telemedicine for the prevention and treatment of youth suicide by connecting widely separated and often isolated programs of varying sizes together into a network of support. For example, small clinics would need to develop separate contracts for services such as child and adult psychiatric support, but the TBHCE is able to provide more cost-effective specialty care conveniently located within the clinic patients utilize for services. Such a system could provide 24/7 access to emergency and routine behavioral health service in any setting with adequate telecommunications service and appropriately trained staff.

The TBHCE also provides opportunities for mutual provider support. For example, currently when psychiatric providers are on leave or are attending a training conference there are often no direct services available during that time period. Sufficient services could be provided via tele-health connections to improve continuity of care with providers who are familiar with treating AI/AN patients. IHS also encourages families to participate in care through tele-health in circumstances when their youth may be transitioning from a treatment facility or residential program.

Providers with particular specialty interests can also share their skills and knowledge across a broad area even if they themselves are located in an isolated location by videoconferencing, providing clinical supervision and working with multidisciplinary teams. Universities providing distance-based learning opportunities have demonstrated for years that educational activities can be facilitated by this technology and reduce burn out due to professional isolation. Recruitment also becomes less problematic because providers can readily live and practice out of larger urban or suburban areas and are thus more likely to continue providing service over time.

The TBHCE also provides virtual training to primary care providers, nurses, and behavioral health providers on current and pressing behavioral health topics in an effort to increase the Indian health system's capacity to provide integrated behavioral health care with primary care. In FY 2014, over 8,000 providers received training.

Recruitment and Retention

The rural and remote geographical locations of AI/AN communities present challenges with recruitment and retention of qualified behavioral health providers. Many of the facilities that serve AI/AN populations are in what the Health Resources and Services Administration (HRSA) has designated as health professional shortage areas. [2] The IHS offers financial incentive programs to recruit and retain behavioral health providers. The IHS Loan Repayment Program offers financial support in exchange for a service obligation in IHS-designated facilities upon completion of training and licensure. The IHS Indian Health Professions Scholarship Program is designed for AI/AN recipients entering the healthcare field. The recipients receive full or partial tuition support and a monthly stipend in exchange for a service obligation upon completion of training and appropriate licensure for placement within IHS-designated facilities located in designated shortage areas. The Indians into Psychology grant provides funding to colleges and universities for the purpose of developing and maintaining American Indian psychology career recruitment pro-

---

[2] See: Health Resources and Services Administration Shortage Designation: Health Professional Shortage Areas and Medically Underserved Areas/Populations. Available at: *www.hrsa.gov/shortage/find*

grams to encourage AI/AN students to enter the behavioral or mental health field. Recipients of the program receive tuition, fees, and a monthly stipend. Upon graduation with a Ph.D., these professionals are placed within IHS-designated facilities.

The National Health Service Corps (NHSC), administered by HRSA, has both a scholarship program and a loan repayment program. The NHSC adds another source of service-obligated providers to IHS, Tribal, and Urban Indian health programs, including behavioral health professionals. IHS and HRSA collaborated to increase the numbers of IHS, Tribal, and Urban Indian health program sites that are eligible for assignment of NHSC personnel. The NHSC Loan Repayment Program is another opportunity for behavioral health providers to serve in communities with limited access to care and have their student loans repaid.

Conclusion

Suicide prevention needs to be addressed in the comprehensive, coordinated way outlined in the National Strategy for Suicide Prevention. No one agency or one approach will solve the tragedy of suicide in AI/AN communities. Suicide is complex and thus has many factors that must be considered. Reducing the number of suicides requires the engagement and commitment of people in many sectors in and outside government. IHS is committed to being a partner in the response to end Native youth suicides. As a central provider of health care for American Indians and Alaska Natives, we must do better in reaching youth with behavioral health and other help they need. We want to work with you to get us closer to the Zero Suicide goal. We all recognize that the challenges faced by Native youth run deep—we must all work together in offering them hope for a better future.

The CHAIRMAN. Thank you so much, Mr. McSwain.

Next we have C.J. Clifford, Council Member from Pine Ridge, South Dakota. I note that President Steele is not with us because he fell ill. Please give him our very best.

Councilman Clifford.

STATEMENT OF HON. COLLINS "C.J." CLIFFORD, TRIBAL COUNCIL MEMBER, OGLALA SIOUX TRIBE

Mr. CLIFFORD. I would like to say top of the afternoon to you, Chairman Barrasso and members of the Committee. Thank you for having me here today.

My name is C.J. Clifford, Council Member for the Oglala Sioux Tribe. I am here in place of our tribal president, John Yellow Bird Steele, who fell ill. President Steele was very disappointed that he could not attend this important hearing.

Between the week before Christmas and today, the Oglala Sioux Tribe has lost 14, to update you with numbers, young people to suicide. According to the Indian Health Service, 176 of our youth attempted suicide in that same period. The IHS treated 229 more who had suicidal ideas with plans and intent to carry it out.

Though there is some overlap with IHS, our Tribe's Sweetgrass Suicide Prevention Project served 276 young people exhibiting suicidal behavior. These are our children and we cannot bear to lose any more. When we lose one child, it hurts the spirit and soul of every one of our people. I hope the hearing today results in action from Congress to assist in saving the lives of our youth.

President Steele issued a proclamation in February 2015 declaring a state of emergency on the Pine Ridge Reservation due to high incidence of suicide of our youth. I would like to submit this for the record. This is the second declaration since 2010. We are struggling and need to get resources to get in front of this problem.

Our biggest challenge is to combat the hopelessness of our youth. We also need to combat the growing normalcy of suicide. Some children speak openly about suicide or discuss methods or stories at the school or on social media.

To reiterate the story you mentioned earlier, this year one of the youth pastors on our reservation received a tip there would be a group suicide that day. He went to the site and found ropes hanging from the trees. Thankfully, no one had hanged themselves but the youth had begun to gather. This intervention saved them at this time.

Feelings of hopelessness are compounded by the reality of living on Pine Ridge. Our poverty rate is more than 50 percent, our unemployment is above 70 percent and 60 percent of our students do not graduate high school. Life expectancy is around 50 years of age compared to the U.S. average of 79 years.

The suicide rate is twice the national average. The latest cluster of suicides is almost unprecedented. Our children have the outlook that things may not get better for them, that they are destined to suffer the same history and injustice as our ancestors.

Black Elk said the nation's circle was broken by Wounded Knee; 125 years later, we are still trying to heal. Just for your information, I am a direct descendent of Black Elk, the holy man.

We have asked IHS to deploy behavioral health professionals. We have asked them to provide debriefing, education and individual assessments and to work with our schools. We have also asked them to begin home visits for youth treated for suicidal ideation, mental health problems or attempted suicide.

IHS has begun to help us but there is so much work that needs to be done. We realize that IHS is struggling to provide adequate services nationwide due to insufficient funding but we are faced with urgent problems in need of immediate attention and assistance.

Congress can help us in concrete ways. Immediate steps include: one, to encourage the Secretary to come out to Pine Ridge for a youth suicide prevention summit and create a task force devoted to accessing Federal resources for suicide prevention and intervention; two, to establish a school-based community so students can have access to counselors at their schools; three, to provide $240,000 through SAMSHA, HRSA or elsewhere to install Tele-Health in our schools; four, establish and fund a Department of Labor youth opportunity program on the Pine Ridge Reservation and make opportunities to provide children with safe havens; five, to immediately provide surplus Federal housing to address our severely overcrowded housing situation which places significant stress on our children.

There are also fundamental overarching steps Congress can take to help us. These are detailed in our written testimony.

I will be glad to answer any questions.

[The prepared statement of Mr. Yellow Bird Steele follows:]

PREPARED STATEMENT OF HON. JOHN YELLOW BIRD STEELE, PRESIDENT, OGLALA
SIOUX TRIBE

Since December, we have lost eleven young people on the Pine Ridge Reservation to suicide.

At least another 176 of our youth attempted it in that period, according to the Indian Health Service, and it treated 229 more with suicidal ideation with plans and intent to carry it out. The Tribe's Sweetgrass Suicide Prevention Project made contact with 276 of our youth exhibiting suicidal behaviors.

We simply cannot bear to lose any more of our children. We must work harder to show them that were are proud of them, that we love and understand them, and that we are there to support them through their hard times; we must demonstrate to our children that they make us happy. Our youth are our future, and therefore are sacred; whenever we lose one child, it hurts the spirit and soul of every one of our people.

On February 17, 2015, I issued a proclamation declaring a state of emergency on our Pine Ridge Reservation due to the high incidence of suicide of our native youth. This is our second such declaration since 2010. We are struggling. We simply do not have the resources to get out in front of this problem, and are working to do everything we can to keep up. Chairman Barrasso, Vice Chairman Tester, and Members of the Committee, thank you for inviting me here today to discuss the prevention of Native youth suicide. There are few topics as urgent as this one, and fewer that are as hard to discuss. I hope this hearing today results in action from this Congress to assist us in saving the lives of our youth. There is no more fundamental way to honor our treaties and the trust responsibility than to ensure the well-being of our young people. They are the future of our Tribe.

One of the most harrowing stories from this epidemic was covered in the New York Times on May 1, 2015. A youth pastor on our Reservation received word that some of our young people had planned a group suicide. The pastor sped to the place it was planned, and found many ropes hanging from the trees. Thankfully he arrived before any children attempted to hang themselves, but found a group of teens had begun to congregate. The pastor prayed with and counseled them on the spot, undoubtedly saving many lives in the process. We can relay stories like this, as horrible as they are, but it is impossible for us to put into words the emotion of seeing a group of friends and family visiting the home of a child who recently took her own life, or to somehow describe the feeling when you see the mother of one of these children doing her best to carry on her day to day life with a wounded spirit. Worst of all, we cannot replace what was missing from the hearts of our lost children.

The Pine Ridge Reservation Suffers from Chronic Poverty and a Sense of Hopelessness

The causes of suicide are not easily defined, nor can we point to just one. What we do know is that we have to meet this threat from every angle. Such a comprehensive approach is challenging anywhere, but the difficulty is compounded by the pervasive problems found on our Reservation like unemployment, overcrowded housing, substandard or unavailable health care, alcoholism and drug abuse, sexual and mental abuse, poor access to food and heat, crumbling schools, and having inadequate access to counseling or mental health resources.

We are also beset with a great deal of violence against our women and children, particularly domestic violence. While we do not have precise statistics about such instances, one of our women's shelter reports 1,300 instances of domestic violence in the last year, while our Department of Public Safety reports 470 prosecuted cases in 2014. We know not all instances are reported or prosecuted, so these numbers are low compared to reality, but are still far too high for our people. This is a cause of great alarm on our Reservation, and we have been attempting to cease such incidents for years. We have made headway, but we are challenged by not only the above factors, but also the fact that we have very little funding for policing from the BIA or funding for our tribal courts from DOJ. The BIA has taken more than 15 years to design the Kyle Justice Center on the eastern part of our Reservation, and it is still not complete. Even with the new special domestic violence jurisdiction and powers under the Tribal Law and Order Act we are prevented from exercising our rightful authority as sovereigns due to unfunded requirements passed by Congress. These limitations prevent us from fully intervening in this parallel crisis for our Tribe.

Nearly 40,000 of our members reside on our Reservation, yet we have just a handful of mental health professionals. Our school counselors, when there are school counselors, are overwhelmed and our social support networks are taxed to their limits. All of this is taking place in a backdrop of a community afflicted. Our real unemployment rate is more than 75%; our school dropout rate is over 60%, and our per-capita income is below $7,000 a year -- 15% of the National average and well, well below the poverty line. Our suicide rate is more than twice the national average.

The poverty on my Reservation—the root cause of these problems—is overwhelming, and we are victims of all the social ills that accompany chronic, severe poverty, including the shortest life expectancy of anywhere in the Western Hemisphere other than Haiti. The adults on my Reservation have little hope, and their children see that every day. There are too few bright spots for our people. Just this spring there were heavy rains and flooding on the Reservation; many of our people lost their homes or property and many of our roads were destroyed. Events like this combined with the backdrop of our everyday lives create despair that is very difficult to see through.

This list of troubles is not complete, of course, and even reciting these causes is exhausting for us to do when we weigh these problems in one hand, and the resources and manpower in the other. There is an imbalance. I talk about them, however, to paint the picture that my people see everyday. A sunny day with a breeze coming over the prairie grass and winding through the Badlands is paradise to any visitor to our Reservation, but for our children, such beauty is obscured by the heavy emotional weight they carry and the ominous outlook that things may not get better for them, that they are destined to suffer the same history and injustices our ancestors suffered. The commitment of our people working to combat these feelings and struggles is second to none, but we are restricted by the lack of resources to address all the contributing factors on our Reservation that result in hopelessness in our children.

We face many challenges, but none is a priority more than instilling a sense of hope in our young people. We are worried that the recent surge in suicides is contagious among our youth, with each incident potentially encouraging others. We also have to combat drug trafficking and alcoholism. We are working to instill cultural values in our youth as a result, but then must address incidents like 57 of our best and brightest students attending a semi-pro hockey game as a reward for their achievements, only to have beer poured on them from a VIP box and being told to "go back to the rez." Helping children as young as eight cope with such an incident is hard enough, but then we had to try to explain to them why our regional newspaper implied it was the children's own fault that they suffered this indignity. Worse, our people look around the Reservation and see neglect by the United States, our trustee and Treaty partner, whose obligations to honor its promises is not minimized by its past failure to do so. The institutions that others in the country can look to for fairness, pride, and investment are sources of disappointment and oppression for Indian people. These are the kinds of obstacles we face.

None of this is new. The United States Commission on Civil Rights detailed the conditions in Indian Country, federal spending, and the trust responsibility in its 2003 report *A Quiet Crisis*. The report decried the low level of appropriations for Indian programs in the face of growing unmet needs from broken promises by the U.S. Government. The Report found that "the anorexic budget of the IHS can only lead one to deduce that less value is placed on Indian health than that of other populations." The Report also clearly stated that trust fulfillment is a civil right for Native people. Congress did not follow through on the Report's recommendations. We need this Committee and this Congress to uphold that civil right: the trust responsibility.

The Government Must Assist Us in Concrete Ways

We can all read the articles and the statistics, but I come here today to seek assistance with the kinds of things we hardly hear about except in our conversations in places like this Committee. Our discussions must spread beyond these four walls, and our requests cannot fall on deaf ears.

We are encouraged by the meeting we had just last week on June 18 with representatives from the Indian Health Service, Administration for Native Americans, Substance Abuse and Mental Health Services Administration, Housing and Urban Development and the Bureau of Indian Affairs to work on addressing this issue. During that meeting, I presented the attached letter to Assistant Secretary for Indian Affairs Kevin Washburn and explained that there are many factors that contribute to our youth's despair. It is the totality of the environment in which they live. If you put an animal in a cage with clean water and water laced with drugs and nothing else, over time that animal will go for the water laced with drugs and do so until it dies. The environment is just too barren, too negative, and the drugged water lets it cope and forget. If you put some food in that cage, place some toys in that cage, pet the animal from time to time and pay it attention, the animal would go for the clean water because he is healthy, safe, and well treated and hopes that life will continue. Even with the loving parents we have on our Reservation, the totality of our youths' surroundings is analogous to that barren, sparse, negative cage. It does not have to be this way; we need to give our youth hope. The federal officials in the meeting last week agreed that we must do what we can to provide hope for our children.

We are also gratified to report that the White House has responded to at least part of our requests, and have provided the Pine Ridge School—a BIB-run school—with $218,000 to help prevent suicide and to help our students and teachers who are traumatized by suicide to heal and recover. The source of the funds is the Department of Education's Project School Emergency Response to Violence grant aid program. The school will use these funds to hire additional counselors and social workers throughout the summer session and in the next school year. This is a good start, but it is just a start to what we need. This is only one of our schools out of 14 schools. Our other schools need these resources also.

Another important aspect to combatting this epidemic is the creation of jobs and economic self-sufficiency. To do so aims directly at the hopelessness that appears to pervade the feelings of our young people. This was not only one of our main requests in my declaration of emergency in February, but has been a constant refrain from the Oglala Lakota Nation. We need support from this Congress to develop infrastructure on the Pine Ridge Reservation that will promote long-term economic self-sufficiency on the Reservation to create permanent jobs to help prevent the causes of this crisis.

We have asked the IHS to deploy Behavioral Health professional to assist us with suicide prevention and intervention. We have asked the IHS hospital to provide debriefing, education, and individual assessment on our youth affected by suicide and to work with our schools to intervene. We also asked the IHS to begin home visits to all homes with youth treated for suicidal ideation, mental health problems, or for attempted suicide. We have not yet seen these services from our trustee. While we realize the IHS is struggling to provide adequate services nationwide due to insufficient funding from Congress, we are faced with a brutally urgent problem, and need immediate assistance.

There are ways this Committee can help us immediately.

1. **Fulfill the United States Government's treaty obligations and fully fund programs.**
   The United States Government's failure to fulfill its treaty obligations to the Oglala Sioux

Tribe in the federal appropriation process is long-standing. It must be remedied. Treaty funding, initially funded by treaty appropriations, are now provided in lump sum program dollars to federal agencies which in turn divide those program dollars up among all tribes, treaty and non-treaty tribes. Consequently, these agencies are short-changing the Tribe in treaty guaranteed services including economic development, education, health, law and order, and others. We see the Government unjustly funding the Tribe at less than 60% of actual need. Treaty benefits are mandatory contractual legal obligations (not entitlements).They should not be subject to sequestration.

The United States Government has a fiduciary trust responsibility under the treaties to protect tribal/Indian property, land, rights and provide resources. Today's Government funding should be protected and guaranteed quid pro quo treaty benefits. Treaties are the supreme law of the land. As U.S. Supreme Court Justice Hugo Black said in 1960, "Great Nations, like great men, should keep their word."

Before the Budget Reform Act and sequestration were considered, the BIA, BIE and IHS Indian programs serving my people were already operating at less than 60% of actual need. So, while we strongly support the funding proposals submitted by the President for those Agencies, as a starting point, we need Congress to understand what the President's proposal really does. After factoring in the unfunded increased costs and increased service population since 2000, and the money taken as a result of sequestration, the President's proposals (according to BIA's own numbers) merely put most of our programs back to just below what we were receiving in FY 2012.

For example, the President's proposed increase of $70 million for Referred Health Care actually consists of: $35 million for actual FY 2016 inflation, $8.3 million for actual FY 2016 documented population growth, and $1.2 to fund the new facility at Yuma. The remaining monies fund: (1) a combined total of 980 additional admissions which divided among the 566 federally recognized tribes, is less than 2 additional admissions per tribe; (2) a combined total of 19,800 new outpatient visits which equates to 3 more outpatient visits per month per tribe, and (3) a combined total of 1,210 new patient trips, which equates to just over 2 more trips per year/per tribe. Every program in the IHS budget has similar shortfalls. Housing efforts only fund 30 to 40 units a year when 100 times that many are needed to alleviate overcrowding. We talk about numbers here in Washington, but in Pine Ridge, these are people. If they cannot access the services they need and that they deserve, it makes it all the much harder to convince them that they are a priority and have value.

2. **Provide Emergency Funding for Substance Abuse, Suicide Prevention, and Mental Health Care.** The suicide emergency at Pine Ridge is dire. It, however, is not unknown either in our history or throughout the history of Indian Country at large. There are multiple avenues for providing funding that already exist, whether they are in the IHS, the Health Resources and Services Administration, or at SAMHSA. The Indian Health Care Improvement Act Reauthorization created a tribal behavioral and mental health grant within SAMHSA that has received only small amounts of funding each year—and only then on a competitive basis. The amount of funding provided could be used up by a small handful of tribes, yet all tribes need such services in substantial amounts.

Congress can also look to existing programs like the Garret Lee Smith Suicide Prevention Program (SAMSHA / Center for Mental Health Services); the Gathering of Native Americans program (SAMHSA), Assessing and Managing Suicide Risk training (SAMHSA / Suicide Prevention Resource Center); Rural Mental Health First Aid (HRSA); the Bullying Prevention Initiative (HRSA), the Methamphetamine and Suicide Prevention Initiative (IHS), and many other program for new and existing avenues of getting funding and services to tribes. There simply needs to be a federal commitment to addressing this need, as we, on Pine Ridge, have no further resources.

3. **Commit to Economic Development and Infrastructure on the Pine Ridge Reservation.** Improving economic development is not an easy task, given that it takes a multi-pronged effort. However, the government's responsibility for fulfilling its treaty obligations in this area is just as important as it is in other areas. Congress must provide full funding for Indian education, including the improvement or rebuilding of our schools so our children have safe, warm, and up-to-date learning spaces. Congress must empower tribal people to pursue their treaty rights, which involves the return of land, wildlife management, and support for agriculture (including industrial hemp farming, for which the Department of Justice and the Drug Enforcement Agency has refused to allow our tribal members to undertake, despite the fact that hemp is not marijuana and marijuana is banned on the Reservation). The United States government should take steps to directly employ our people on the Reservation for these efforts and facilitate other job opportunities for our members.

It is also critical for the government to provide Tribes their fair share of infrastructure funding. The Committee is well aware that federal aid highways provide only a small fraction of the funding needed for us to bring our roads and bridges up to standard. BIA road maintenance funding is only at 13% of the need. Our Reservation buildings are falling apart, and our clinics are substandard. The Mni Wiconi Project, which serves our communities with a safe and adequate water supply, needs to be completed as Congress intended; this includes upgrading and transferring the community water systems.

It may not seem like infrastructure is an important part of suicide prevention, but I urge you to come to my Reservation and see for yourself. If you look around you will see crumbling bridges, pot-holed or washed out roads or what used to be paved roads crumbling back to gravel, or schools with leaky roofs and inadequate heat. What would you think? Our children see this and think, "We're not worth the effort." That is unacceptable to us, and should be unacceptable to everyone. We cannot fathom why such neglect is allowed to continue. We need to reverse it for the sake of our Nation.

4. **Remove Jurisdictional Restrictions and Fund Tribal Law Enforcement and Justice.** Protecting our people from crime and intervening in domestic violence is critical to our efforts to reduce the rate of suicide on the Reservation. Today, the expanded jurisdiction provisions of the Violence Against Women Act (VAWA) and Tribal Law and Order Act (TLOA) are not working for the majority of the large land based tribes. Congress and the Administration never told us that if we wanted to expand our jurisdiction over domestic violence or serious offenders, we had to find our own funding. Juxtapose the expanded

jurisdiction provisions of these two Acts with the BIA budgets for Courts and Law enforcement and you can see that the VAWA and TLOA's expanded jurisdiction provisions are unfulfilled promises.

There have been funding increases in law enforcement over the last few years. However, those increases have not provided us with an increase in officers. Today, Pine Ridge is still short 60 officers from the minimum 110 that the BIA itself, says we need. Our officers are exhausted and morale is at an all-time low.

Our tribal courts also need funding increases. Adding more funding to law enforcement without increasing funding for our courts simply shifts the problem from one side to the other. TLOA and VAWA have created new expectations for our members. We need the Federal government to ensure that our tribal courts and law enforcement programs can fulfill those expectations. Simply put, we need the resources to shore up our police force and make necessary changes to our courts to ensure our judiciary systems work effectively.

BIA's failure to complete the design for our Kyle Justice Center is one of the most pressing problems facing our community. This Justice Center has been at the top of the BIA's construction priority list for over fifteen years. It is not a long term "detention" facility, where alternatives to incarceration can be considered. It is a short term holding facility, a court and a 911 center for the eastern side of our Reservation. This will be the place that our law enforcement will take violent and dangerous persons awaiting arraignment or trial. We need a place to put individuals until sentencing or alternative treatment arrangements can be handed down by our tribal court. Letting offenders back out into the streets just increases the likelihood of violence. We need the resources for officers, courts, and facilities to stanch the cycle of abuse and harm on our lands.

5. **Focus on Education and our Schools.** I mentioned earlier the infusion of funding for the Pine Ridge School to hire counselors for the faculty and students. That is an important step towards improving the place where our youth spend much of their time: our schools. The state of schools in Indian Country is a national disgrace, and the Bureau of Indian Education (BIE) is moving at a glacial pace to replace facilities and improve operations. Congress has failed to appropriate sufficient funding to allow schools to both maintain and function day-to-day, forcing our communities to choose one at the expense of the other. Now, the BIE is engaged in a reform effort that they say is "school improvement," but really only is a shift in its own bureaucracy. School Improvement will come when our schools receive their deserved direct funding to hire teachers and staff that will be able to impart culture, knowledge, and self-esteem to our youth. We applaud the Congress's move to fully fund maintenance at our schools, but increased funding for operations, reduced bureaucratic requirements by the BIE, full funding for tribal colleges, and immediate funding for improvement or reconstruction of our school facilities is also required. Our best chance to reach youth is at school, and we must be able to make school a beacon of hope for them.

6. **Follow Through On Commitments.** As I said earlier, we met with many government officials last week to discuss this crisis on my Reservation. Representatives of HHS, IHS, and the BIA all agreed that action was needed. The question now is when will that action take place? My Reservation has also been recently designated a Promise Zone by the President, a program designed to accelerate economic mobility in high poverty communities. While a Promise Zone designation does not come with money, the program is designed to help cut red tape, and to provide us with professional assistance on grant and loan applications to help us complete our sustainable development plan in housing and education. Our federal partners must assist us in meeting these goals; our federal partners include Congress.

A bright spot for us in this struggle is the Tribe's Sweet Grass Suicide Prevention Project, which was designed by the Tribe to address youth suicide and prevention on the Reservation. As with all of our programs, however, the Sweet Grass Project's funding is in jeopardy. The program's staff works 24 hours a day to be there for our youth in crisis, and work proactively to prevent suicide and self-harm by integrating healing practices based on our Lakota culture and history. The Lakota Culture is very important in suicide prevention in order to be effective: one primary aspect is *Wowaunsila* (having compassion for the people). Another is *Wokigna* (comforting people when they are experiencing the psychic pain that prompts them to commit suicide). Another is *Wazila* (a Lakota cultural way of using sweet grass or sage to purify an area) before one offers a *Wochekiya* (an appeal to the creator and the spirits for assistance during a difficult time).

Sweet Grass Project staff and volunteers at all times are on call to help anyone who needs for assistance in a crisis, and they are constantly seeking to engage our community proactively to avert tragedies before they happen. The Project also helps train "first responders," since coaching people not to panic when they are in a suicidal situation is important, because they need to stay with the individual until help arrives. This is where the cultural value *Woohitika* (bravery, finding the courage within oneself to stay calm during this critical time) plays its most important role. Most people on the Pine Ridge Reservation who express ideation are under the influence of alcohol or drugs, and cannot always help themselves. This is why it is important to get others involved to help: *Tiwahe* (the immediate family), *Tiospaye* (the extended family), *Ospaye* (the community), *Chanksa yuha* (law enforcement) and tribal programs. All of these play an important role in our efforts, and it is critical that we have the resources to develop and sustain the relationships between them to help prevent suicide and suicidal ideation.

We remain committed to beating the epidemic of youth suicide on the Pine Ridge Reservation, and we hope that you respond to our requests for assistance. Please do not hesitate to contact me if you have any questions.

Attachment

Oglala Sioux Tribe
Office of the President

MEMORANDUM

TO: Kevin Washburn, Assistant Secretary for Indian Affairs

FR: John Yellowbird Steele, President *John Yellow Bird Steele*
    Oglala Sioux Tribe

Re: Treaty Rights, Sovereignty & Jurisdiction; Criminal Justice; Suicide Prevention;
Roads and Infrastructure; Health Care, Education and Housing.

Date: June 18, 2015

OGLALA SIOUX TRIBE: STATISTICS

The Oglala Sioux Tribe is the largest tribe of the Great Sioux Nation, with
more than 47,000 tribal members and an extensive reservation, which spans more
than 2.8 million acres and almost 4,000 square miles is larger than the States of
Delaware and Rhode Island combined.

The U.S. Census reports: Oglala Lakota County, on the western side of the
Pine Ridge Reservation, is the third poorest county in the Nation, measured in per
capita income. In Oglala Lakota County, more than 55% of our people live below the
poverty line compared to 14.5% nationwide, and the average per capita income is
about $8,768 compared with the average of $25,740 for South Dakota and more
than $28,000 nationwide. We have an unemployment rate of well over 70%, and
educational attainment is low: we have a high school dropout rate of over 60%, and we
have only 11.8% of the adult population having attained a bachelor's degree
compared with more than 26% statewide and 28.8% nationwide. More than 38% of
Oglala Lakota County people are under 18 years old.

Housing, health care, education, public safety, infrastructure, and economic
development are all impacted by poverty on our Reservation. Time and again, BIA
and IHS budgets have fallen short to meet our many needs. Until the United States
honors its treaty obligations and provides adequate base, non-competitive, funding,
progress on our Reservation will continue to be elusive. We strive to improve our
members' lives, but we cannot do that without infrastructure, safe housing, quality
education, proper healthcare, and economic development.

We have a suicide epidemic on Pine Ridge: Several young people -- including a 12-year-old -- have committed suicide on the Pine Ridge Reservation. There have been more than 140 attempts in the past year. (See New York Times, May 2, 2015 Pine Ridge Indian Reservation Struggles with Suicides Among its Young.) More needs to be done to meet the United States trust responsibility to provide mental health care to our Indian people, especially our youth. We need the Federal government to act to address our epidemic. I issued a proclamation and declared a state of emergency. It declares that Congress should support a bill to develop infrastructure on the Pine Ridge Reservation that will promote sustainable economic self-sufficiency on the Reservation and create permanent jobs. The lack of jobs is the real cause of abject poverty, alcohol and drug abuse, crime and health care issues like suicide.

Recently, we have had melting snow, heavy rains and flooding. The Oglala Sioux Tribe has had to declare a Flood Emergency and requested FEMA help. Naturally, we need help from the BIA as well. People have lost their houses and property. We have had roads and bridges wash out and the impact is several million dollars. We need those roads and bridges repaired, so our people can travel safely on our reservation roads. We will show the impact of this flooding as we travel the Pine Ridge Reservation.

TREATY RIGHTS, INDIAN SOVEREIGNTY AND TRIBAL JURISDICTION

Through the 1803 Louisiana Purchase Treaty, the United States laid claim to the Louisiana Territory, including North and South Dakota, subject to the existing rights of Native Nations. The Treaty, in Article VI, provides for a continuing treaty relationship between the United States and Indian nations and tribes: "The United States promise to execute Such treaties and articles as may have been agreed between Spain and the tribes and nations of Indians until by mutual consent of the United States and the said tribes or nations other Suitable articles Shall have been agreed upon." (France had recently acquired its Louisiana claim from Spain).

The Oglala Sioux Tribe has a treaty relationship with the United States, including the 1815 Treaty, 1825 Treaty, 1836 Treaty, 1851 Treaty and 1868 Sioux Nation Treaty. The 1851 Fort Laramie Treaty acknowledges the original territory of the Oglala Sioux Tribe, including the Black Hills of South Dakota.

Chief Red Cloud fought the 1866-1868 Powder River War to protect the Black Hills and the Powder River Country. At the end of the War, the United States entered the 1868 Sioux Nation Treaty, promising that "all war between the parties shall forever cease" and pledging its "honor" to keep the peace.

- **Great Sioux Nation Reservation:** The Great Sioux Reservation was reserved as the *"permanent home"* of the Oglala Sioux Tribe and other Lakota Oyate "commencing on the east bank of the Missouri River" and along the lower water from the 46th parallel of longitude in the north down to the Nebraska state line and west to the 104th degree of longitude west from Greenwich ... then back to the point of beginning. Thus, the Great Sioux

Reservation encompassed all of western South Dakota, including the Black Hills and the southern most strip of North Dakota west of the Missouri River.

- **Unceded Indian Territory:** 44 million acres of unceded Indian territory from "north of the North Platte River and east of the summits of the Big Horn Mountains shall be held and considered to be unceded Indian territory ... ·and no white person shall be permitted to settle upon or occupy any portion of the same; or without the consent of the Indians ... to pass through the same and it is further agreed by the United States that ... after the conclusion of peace with ... the Sioux Nation, the military posts ... shall be abandoned...."

- *Sovereignty and Self-Government:* The 1868 Sioux Nation Treaty expressly reserves the original, inherent sovereignty of the Sioux Nation and the Oglala Sioux Tribe. In *Ex Parte Crow Dog,* 109 U.S. 556 (1883) the Supreme Court held that Crow Dog could not be hanged by the United States for the murder of Spotted Tail because the 1868 Treaty reserved self-government rights. As the Court explained, "[t]he pledge to secure to these people, with whom the United States was contracting as a distinct political body, an orderly government ... necessarily implies ... that among the arts of civilized life, which it was the very purpose of all these arrangements to introduce and naturalize among them, was the highest and best of all,—that of self-government, the regulation by themselves of their own domestic affairs, the maintenance of order and peace among their own members by the administration of their own laws and customs."

THE BLACK HILLS WERE STOLEN IN VIOLATION OF THE 1868 SIOUX NATION TREATY AND THE CONSTITUTION AND THE PRESIDENT SHOULD MEET WITH SIOUX NATION TRIBAL AND TRADITIONAL LEADERS TO DISCUSS MOVING FORWARD WITH JUSTICE IN THE BLACK HILLS

In 1876—77, the United States made war on the Sioux Nation in violation of the 1868 Treaty, sending out Custer to attack the Lakota, Cheyenne and Arapaho at the Little Big Horn, Crook to the Rosebud, McKenzie to Wolf Mountain, and Mills at Slim Buttes, the United States unconstitutionally stole the Black Hills from the Sioux Nation without compensation.

Concerning President Grant's "duplicity" in refusing to uphold the 1868 Treaty and the pattern of duress used by the United States in the attempt to force the cession of the Black Hills through starvation, the Supreme Court explained in *United States v. Sioux Nation,* 448 U.S. 371 (1980) that: "A more ripe and rank case of dishonorable dealings will never, in all probability, be found in our history...."

On August 23, 2012, the Great Plains Tribal Chairman's Association vote to request a meeting with President Obama and the Sioux Nation on the Black Hills and I sent the attached Letter to President Obama requesting a meeting on the Black

Hills with our Sioux Nation tribal leaders and traditional leaders. We would like to renew our request that during or before the next White House Tribal Nations Meeting, President Obama should meet with our Sioux Nation tribal and traditional leaders to discuss a process for moving forward towards justice on the Black Hills.

REQUEST: GIVE PRIORITY TO INDIAN TRIBES WITH FULL CRIMINAL AND CIVIL JURISDICTION OVER OUR INDIAN LANDS AND TAKE INTO ACCOUNT SERVICE POPULATIONS AND LAND AREAS, WHEN BIA ALLOCATES FUNDS FOR TRIBAL CRIMINAL LAW ENFORCEMENT AND TRIBAL COURTS.

The Oglala Sioux Tribe adopted its Constitution and By-Laws pursuant to the Indian Reorganization Act and exercises law enforcement authority throughout the entire 1889 Act boundaries of the Pine Ridge Indian Reservation, including Oglala Lakota County, southern Jackson (former Washabaugh) County, and Bennet County. Under Article IV, Powers of the Council, Section 1(K), the Oglala Sioux Tribal Council has authority to:

> To promulgate and enforce ordinances, governing the conduct of persons on the Pine Ridge Indian Reservation, and providing for the maintenance and order and the administration of justice by establishing a reservation court and defining its duties and powers.

The Oglala Sioux Tribe Constitution establishes a tribal court system: "The judicial power of the Oglala Sioux Tribe in one Supreme Court and in inferior tribal courts established by the Tribal Council.... The judicial power shall extend to all cases arising in law and equity, arising under the Oglala Sioux Tribe Constitution, the laws of the Oglala Sioux Tribe, or to all persons and property within the jurisdiction of the Oglala Sioux Tribe...." Oglala Sioux Tribe Constitution, Article V, secs. 1 and 2.

The Oglala Sioux Tribe has boundaries firmly established by the 1868 Sioux Nation Treaty ("absolute and undisturbed use" of "permanent home") and the Act of March 2, 1889. The State of South Dakota has disclaimed jurisdiction over the Pine Ridge Indian Reservation pursuant to the State enabling Act:

> "We, the people of South Dakota ... forever disclaim all right and title to ... all lands ... owned or held by any Indian or Indian tribes; and ... said Indian lands shall remain under the absolute jurisdiction and control of the Congress of the United States...."

State Constitution Preamble and Article XXII Compact with the United States. Accordingly, the State of South Dakota disclaims criminal jurisdiction over Indians on the Pine Ridge Reservation. *See State v. Cummins*, 679 N.W.2d 484 (S.D. Sup. Ct. 2004) (State police have no authority to arrest Indians on Pine Ridge Reservation, distinguishing *Nevada v. Hicks*).

Accordingly, the Oglala Sioux Tribe exercises criminal jurisdiction over all Indians on the Pine Ridge Indian Reservation, 25 U.S.C. sec. 1301 et seq., and tribal police officers respond to all public safety and criminal law enforcement situations. Tribal Police officers are vested as Special Law Enforcement Officers Commissioned by the BIA to enforce Federal laws and stop, detain and transport any non-Indian offenders to Fall River County where appropriate. *United States v. Terry*, 400 F.3d 575 (8th Cir. 2005) (Federal prosecution of fire arm charge; Oglala Sioux tribal police stop, detain, transport of non-Indian offender upheld).

Domestic Violence. Today, the expanded jurisdiction provisions of the Violence Against Women Act (VAWA) and Tribal Law and Order Act (TLOA) are not working for the majority of the large land based tribes. These reservations house the overwhelming majority of on-reservation Indians. Congress and the Administration never told us that if we wanted to expand our jurisdiction over domestic violence or serious offenders, we had to find our own funding. Juxtapose the expanded jurisdiction provisions of these two Acts with the BIA budgets for Courts and Law enforcement and you can see that the VAWA and TLOA's expanded jurisdiction provisions are unfulfilled promises. Additionally, the Great Plains Tribes were the authors of the TOLA provisions calling for detailed studies of law enforcement and court shortages. We included these provisions because we were told that those studies would be utilized to justify additional funding. Instead, there have been lost officers and court dollars since TLOA was passed, because of increased fuel costs, unfunded inflation and sequestration.

There have been funding increases in law enforcement over the last few years. However, those increases have not provided us with an increase in officers. Today, Pine Ridge is still short 60 officers from the minimum 110 that the BIA itself, says we need. Our officers are exhausted and morale is at an all-time low.

Our tribal courts also need funding increases. Often too many of those who are arrested are released because they were not afforded timely due process. Adding more funding to law enforcement without increasing funding for our courts simply shifts the problem from one side to the other. TLOA and VAWA have created new expectations for our members. We need the Federal government to ensure that our tribal courts and law enforcement programs can fulfill those expectations. Simply put, we need the resources to shore up our police force and make necessary changes to our courts to ensure our judiciary systems work effectively.

An action that can be taken at no additional cost to taxpayers would be to move the money that Congress is currently expending on DOJ Indian law enforcement, court and detention grants back to the BIA. By taking this one step, you can eliminate a sizable portion of our law enforcement officer shortage, because you will be placing those funds in the highest priority areas. You will also eliminate the duplicate overhead that you are currently paying, and stop the problems associated with trying to use unreliable DOJ grants to run law enforcement and court programs. Alternatively, DOJ should be authorized to do Public Law 638 contracts, and contract with Interior for administration of those contracts.

BIA's failure to complete the design for our Kyle Justice Center is one of the most pressing problems facing our community. This Justice Center has been at the top of the BIA's construction priority list for over fifteen years. It is not a long term "detention" facility, where alternatives to incarceration can be considered. It is a short term holding facility, a court and a 911 center for the eastern side of our Reservation. This will be the place that our law enforcement will take violent and dangerous persons awaiting arraignment or trial. We need a place to put individuals until sentencing or alternative treatment arrangements can be handed down by our tribal court.

Congress chose to fund the design of this replacement building after it determined that our old building was beyond repair. We initiated that design and as the BIA standards for this building changed, so did the cost of the design work. We now have a design which is 80% complete, at a federal cost of just over $2.4 million, and we need $636,000 to complete that design work. Importantly, if this design does not get finalized this year, the architects involved will not warrant the finished product and some of the plans may need to be changed again. Not finishing this work would be a serious waste of taxpayer dollars. Further, this building, like many other large land based jails and court complexes, is going to cost more to construct than DOJ is authorized to spend. This is the reason that the large Tribes have been calling for a re-opening of the BIA Justice Services Construction Program: to address these large facility needs. The only way this critically needed facility and others like it are going to be built is with multi-year funding, which DOJ is not authorized to provide. Will you work with us to find a way to complete this design and build this critically needed building?

Also, we request you work to reinstate the $620,000 in education funding taken from the juvenile detention budget in FY 2012. This funding is desperately needed to provide educational services to detained and incarcerated youth at 24 BIA-funded juvenile detention facilities, including the Kiyuksa O'Tipi Reintegration Center on Pine Ridge. We urge the reinstatement of these monies to address the needs of some of our most vulnerable youth.

WHITE HOUSE NATIVE NATIONS POLICY

We must always remember that Indian nations and tribes were independent sovereigns prior to the formation of the United States. Through treaties, the United States entered into nation-to-nation agreements with Indian nations and tribes that acknowledge our original, inherent sovereign authority over our members and our territory. The Constitution enshrines the earliest Indian treaties and authorized more than 350 Indian treaties, including the 1868 Sioux Nation Treaty.

President Obama has made great progress with the establishment of the White House Council on Native American Affairs under Executive Order No. 13647 (2013), which provides:

To honor treaties and recognize tribes' inherent sovereignty and right to self-government under U.S. law, it is the policy of the United States to promote the development of prosperous and resilient tribal communities, including by:

(a) promoting sustainable economic development, particularly energy, transportation, housing, other infrastructure, entrepreneurial, and workforce development to drive future economic growth and security;

(b) supporting greater access to, and control over, nutrition and healthcare, including special efforts to confront historic health disparities and chronic diseases;

(c) supporting efforts to improve the effectiveness and efficiency of tribal justice systems and protect tribal communities;

(d) expanding and improving lifelong educational opportunities for American Indians and Alaska Natives, while respecting demands for greater tribal control over tribal education,

The Secretary of the Interior chairs the White House Council on Native American Affairs. To make the White House Council an operational part of government, the Council should meet on a quarterly basis with Tribal Governments and undertake to help resolve interagency issues with identified by tribal leaders.

In his speeches, President Obama has often referred to Indian nations and tribes as Native Nations. **TO MAKE PRESIDENT OBAMA'S POLICY LAST INTO THE FUTURE, WE NEED A WHITE HOUSE NATIVE NATIONS POLICY ISSUED THROUGH A NATIVE NATIONS EXECUTIVE ORDER:**

A new Executive Order on Native Nations, which
- Acknowledges Indian nations and tribes as original Native Nations, with sovereign authority over our members and territory;
- Directs Federal Departments and Agencies to defer to Native Nations on matters of internal self-governance and deal with Native Nations on the basis of nation-to-nation relations based upon mutual respect, and mutual consent;
- Directs Federal Departments and Agencies to adhere to the essential principles of the U.N. Declaration on the Rights of Indigenous Peoples, including:
  o Respect and protection for Indian lands and territories;
  o Respect for Indian Self-Determination;
  o Support for Native Education, Health Care, Housing, Economic Development, Transportation and Infrastructure;
  o Respect for Native religions, cultures, and languages; and
  o Respect for Native lifeways.

The Executive Order should direct the White House Council on Native American Affairs to meet quarterly with our Native Nations to discuss intergovernmental concerns on a nation-to-nation, government-to-government basis;

Affirm Executive Order 13175 on Consultation and Coordination with Indian Tribal Governments;

President Obama can leave a legacy of a lasting and meaningful Indian Affairs Policy that equals or exceeds that of his predecessors, including FDR, JFK, Nixon, Reagan, and Clinton, by issuing this new Native Nations.

TREATY APPROPRIATIONS

Our first and foremost concern is the U.S. Government's failure to fulfill its treaty obligations to the Oglala Sioux Tribe in the federal appropriation process. Treaty funding, initially funded by treaty appropriations, are now provided in lump sum program dollars to federal agencies who in turn divide those program dollars up among treaty and non-treaty tribes. Consequently, these agencies are short-changing the Tribe in treaty guaranteed services including economic development, education, health, law and order, and others. We see the Government unjustly funding the Tribe at less than 60% of actual need. Treaty benefits are mandatory contractual legal obligations (not entitlements).They should not be subject to sequestration.

The United States Government has a fiduciary trust responsibility under the treaties to protect tribal/Indian property, land, rights and provide resources. Today's Government funding should be protected and guaranteed quid pro quo treaty benefits. Treaties are the supreme law of the land, As U.S. Supreme Court Justice Hugo Black said in 1960, *"Great Nations, like great men, should keep their word."*

Before the Budget Reform Act and sequestration were considered, the BIA, BIE and IHS Indian programs serving my people were already operating at less than 60% of actual need. So, while we strongly support the funding proposals submitted by the President for those Agencies, as a starting point, we need Congress to understand what the President's proposal really does. After factoring in the unfunded increased costs and increased service population since 2000, and the money taken as a result of sequestration, the President's proposals (according to BIA's own numbers) merely put most of our programs back to just below what we were receiving in FY 2012.

For example, the President's proposed increase of $70 million for Referred Health Care actually consists of: $35 million for actual FY 2016 inflation, $8.3 million for actual FY 2016 documented population growth, and $1.2 to fund the new facility at Yuma. The remaining monies fund: (1) a combined total of 980 additional admissions which divided among the 566 federally recognized tribes, is less than 2 additional admissions per tribe; (2) a combined total of 19,800 new outpatient visits which equates to 3 more outpatient visits per month per tribe, and (3) a combined total of 1,210 new patient trips, which equates to just over 2 more trips per year/per tribe. Every program in the IHS budget has similar shortfalls. We talk about numbers here in Washington, but in Pine Ridge, these are people.

ROADS AND INFRASTRUCTURE

While Congress is talking about cutting spending and sequestering funds, our infrastructure, most of which was built in or before the 1960's, is continuing to fall apart. We have schools, clinics, jails and roads which are beyond repair, yet the federal government keeps appropriating just enough money to add another patch. We have band-aided these items for so long that some of our roads, roofs, furnaces and walls have almost as many patches as they do original surface materials. Indian reservations are in an infrastructure crisis. Unless and until someone comes up with a real plan to rebuild our dilapidated schools, jails, clinics and roads, things will get worse.

We also need a fair share of Federal Highway Trust Funds to address our failing roads. An underlying problem is that our Indian roads programs have never received a reasonable amount of federal gas tax dollars. Permanent re-authorization of the Federal Highway Trust Fund is not before this Subcommittee, but this Subcommittee is left with the problems these funding shortfalls create. Failing roads raise the cost of on-reservation ambulance service, student transportation, law enforcement operations and every other BIA, BIE and IHS program which uses vehicles. It is also adding to our health care costs, because our people are having accidents that never would have happened if we had a safe transportation system. Finally, it is crippling our reservation economic development. In fact, our entire roads system at Pine Ridge was designed to encourage members to leave the reservation for goods and services, not for helping us develop successful on-reservation businesses. Increasing the overall Indian allocation is the only way to solve the problem. The budget for Tribes has been around $26 million for 20 years it should be $160 million a year; the budget doesn't consider maintenance backlog of Tribes.

Current funding is about 13% of need; routine bridge maintenance is not being performed unless it becomes an emergency; snow and ice control can take up to 50% of an annual budget; Tribes feel that the government should fully fund road maintenance and not rely on the tribe's road construction funds to perform road maintenance and Federal Highway Administration construction dollars are supplemental; not in lieu of Tribal Priority Allocations.

The Roads Maintenance Program is responsible for maintenance of 29,500 miles of BIA-owned roads and more than 931 BIA-owned bridges constructed under the Indian Reservation Roads (IRR) program in Indian Country. The TPA funding that Tribes receive will only allow approximately $716.00 per mile for maintenance.

Funding needs to be allocated on a Region by Region basis; with emphasis on the miles of roads, bridges, land base and population. The Tribes of the Great Plains have hundreds of miles of roads to maintain yet in 2010, we were funded at $25 M.

while Alaska was funded at $71.4 million and the Midwest Region received $51.7 M. (a 289 %) increase. Consideration must be given to the differences in each region and to Large & Needy tribes. Indian Reservation Road funding, must be limited for use on the Interior Reservation Roads only. The Great Plains Tribal Chairman's Association supports the new manager amendments to the MAP 21 Highway bill that allows for more equitable distribution of Transportation funding to large land based tribes with more needs and higher inventories. Funding in the legislation barely maintains current funding levels for IRR and needs to be increased to at least $500,000.00.

Economic Development: A special category/consideration is needed for Large and Needy Tribes. Large and Needy Tribes that suffer from severe economic hardships and great challenges to economic development and lack the financial resources and infrastructure to ignite their economies should be targeted for services. The Indian Guaranteed Loan Program must be restored to full funding of at least $10 Million, and labor force and statistics should be reported annually to assist tribes in obtaining formula based funding.

HEALTH CARE

Currently, the IHS funds Indian Health Care at $2750 per Indian patient compared to the U.S. average medical care expenditure of over $7000 per patient. Our Tribe and IHS service unit are still experiencing severe funding shortfalls in this category. This is due to several factors:

- Insufficient facility physicians and other staff, which defers patient treatment until a life-threatening event;
- Delayed services resulting in Life threatening events that are more costly;
- Prior year payments that consume current year funding, resulting in continued funding shortfalls that mean we never get ahead (e.g. Bennett County Hospital)
- A national Program Funding Formula that favors "compacting/contracting regions".

Medical Funding should be based upon an Indian patient's rights to fair medical treatment: One patient, one level of funding just like one person, one vote. Funding should be based on a per patient basis, with adequate funding for facilities. An IHS workgroup devised a formula that now permits those Areas without an inpatient facility to receive additional, off-the-top funding from a 20% pool, and in addition to receiving an Area Allocation from the remaining CHS amounts. We strenuously object to this formula, as we are being penalized for having an understaffed facility.

We ask that you fund the IHS at levels that will help us achieve our stated Tribal and Legislative goals of *100% of Need*. We understand that this task is not one that can be achieved overnight, but your support for a 10-15% increase ($440M to $660M) over the budget request would go a long way towards achieving this objective. We are in need of these amounts to not only maintain current services to our tribal members, but to also fulfill the promises of the recently enacted Indian Health Care Improvement act amendments.

Health Manpower. We are grateful to see that the Health Resources and Services Administration (HRSA) and the IHS have entered into an agreement that will transfer more National Health Service Corp (NHSC) personnel to IHS sites. We ask that these doctors and other professionals be assigned to reservation postings, where the need is the greatest. We do _not_ support the proposed IHS health manpower decrease contained in the IHS budget request and ask that there be a modest 4% increase to this program to keep the scholarship and service obligation pipeline intact.

Indian Health Care Improvement Initiatives. We ask that the Departments support funding to implement:

1. _VA-IHS Partnership Initiative,_ permitting an IHS facility to treat, and bill VA for, an eligible Indian veteran care (which would require the IHS to make the veteran's co-payment in order to recover 80% cost of care); and

2. _Long –Term Care Initiative,_ to establish a much needed-services for our elderly and disabled. We hope this program could include home-based care to help reduce patient travel for minor but necessary services (visiting nurse checkup, medications, physical therapy). Such a program would go a long ways towards ensuring an improved quality of life for some of our most vulnerable, as well as provide our communities with services that other regions and populations take for granted.

Sanitation, Facilities. This is a program area that is vital to maintaining the life of our structures and for improved public health conditions. We oppose the $16M+ Sanitation decrease proposed in the IHS budget request and support the IHS requested amounts for the other facility programs (Construction @ $81.4M, Maintenance and Improvement @ $55.4M, Environmental Support @ $204.3M)

EDUCATION

Thank you for taking an interest in the recent GAO report on our Indian Schools. The Federal Government tells us it wants to "help us" increase our tribal self-sufficiency, but it ignores the biggest tool we have: the improved education of our children. President Obama talks about national efforts to keep more students in college, but at Pine Ridge, I am still trying to keep our sixteen (16) year olds in high school, and give them the self-esteem they need to avoid the ever present threats of alcohol, drugs and suicide. While you work out our failed school construction program, those schools need adequate maintenance monies _and_ adequate operations dollars. Without adequate operations monies for things like heat and electricity, our schools are forced to somehow find monies in the maintenance budget to pay these costs. Thus, our educational facilities go without proper maintenance. The BIA compartmentalizes the budgets for school operations and maintenance, but for those institutions it is all one big problem.

The Great Plains Region has approximately 33 BIE Schools and 1 dormitory, which is 18 % of Tribal Schools Nation-wide. We have about 11,000 students attending BIE schools or 23 % of population for BIE schools nation-wide. The Great Plains have 10 Tribal Colleges on our Reservations. Tribal education in the Great Plains region is at the center of our Priorities and we are proud of our Tribal Schools and our Tribal Colleges. While many Tribes in Different Regions do not have Tribal Schools Tribal Education remains a priority for our Tribes. Overall the Great Plains is the second largest provider of BIE Schools in the Nation with 6 Tribal Education Departments.

Recommendations: Request $156,084,000 for Tribal Education.
-Adequately Fund Tribal Education Departments.
-Promote Tribal Education Department Development of Curriculum.
-Each Region is different, we are not all the same and the same is not equal
-The GPTCA requests full consideration for cultural, political and economic differences
-Fund the Schools before you fund BIE initiatives at the national level.
-Forward Funding under the TCSA and ESEA Should be Held at the Tribal Education Department Level and Reservation Level for investment and not within BIE.
-Enforce 25 U.S.C. § 2011 Government-to-Government "Meaningful" Consultation
-Fully Fund Tribal Colleges and Set Aside Funds from TRIO for tribal colleges.
-Fully fund the BIE school operations and maintenance at 100 %
-Maintain the Tribal Education line Officer at the Local Tribal level
-Restore functions & authority of Indian Education back to the Bureau of Indian Affairs to allow improved cost effectiveness and in keeping with consolidation.
-Increase funding for Construction so all of our tribal schools can be repaired or replaced over the course of the next five years.

WATER: MNI WICONI

The Mni Wiconi Project Act specifically includes that the United States has a trust responsibility to provide safe and adequate water to the Pine Ridge, Rosebud and Lower Brule Indian Reservations. While the Mni Wiconi Project is almost complete, more work is needed to finish the distribution system on the Pine Ridge Reservation. Additionally, the existing community systems, which are a part of the Project, need to be upgraded and transferred into the Oglala Sioux Rural Water Supply System. The Project cannot be considered complete without the upgrade and transfer of these community systems which Congress always intended. Further, without the completion of the Project, the United States cannot fulfill the trust responsibility specifically set forth in the Act. We, therefore, ask that the Administration to support Mni Wiconi Amendment legislation and to engage directly in the interagency effort to address the Project's community systems upgrade issue.

HOUSING: SHORTAGE

Housing is in such short supply at Pine Ridge that multiple families are forced to cram into small trailers, and as many as 18 people have been recorded living in a single home. More money needs to be allocated to the nation's poorest tribes, which don't have enough resources to meet their members' basic needs.

Acquiring land isn't the problem on Pine Ridge; many families there already own property passed down from treaties. What they need is money to build houses. "We have three or four families living in one house," says Paul Iron Cloud, director of the Oglala Sioux Housing Authority. And those overcrowded living conditions affect everything from public health to education. "How do you think you could study with three families in one house?"

Oglala Sioux (Lakota) Housing has built over 2,200 housing units since 1961 but most of that was done before 1996 and the establishment of the Native American Housing Assistance and Self-Determination Act. Sadly in 2015 our housing, and tribal housing on many similarly situated reservations and Alaskan Native communities, is far worse today than 20 years ago. Though NAHASDA provides us and many other tribes and tribal housing entities valuable resources, because of stagnant and reduced funding levels as well as flawed funding allocation methods, we and a large number of other tribes today have the worst housing in the United States.

For at least a generation now, many of our people, infants, elders, vets and families have had to live in housing conditions that no American should have to endure. For these land based tribes, these conditions are also caused by poverty and unemployment rates that in some cases exceed 80 percent. At Pine Ridge and many nearby South Dakota reservations for years now our counties have ranked in the top five in the entire country for poverty and unemployment.

NAHASDA funding levels limit us to building on average no more than 30 to 40 units a year, yet we currently need 4,000 new units and 1,000 homes repaired. The result is that we now have the most overcrowded housing in this country. We have many situations where 3 or 4 families are packed into a single two-bedroom home or a family of six tries to survive in a one bedroom apartment. Overcrowding affects the physical, social and mental state of our people. Schooling is impacted, health conditions suffer and the family unit is impaired. Imagine what it might be like to live with 12 to 16 people in a small home. These housing conditions also fuel our growing tragedies of suicides, sexual abuse, alcoholism, gangs and drug use in many of our communities.

Tribal leaders are most troubled by what these housing conditions do to a child trying to do his or her homework, a young family starting out their married life, our honored vets and our tribal elders who are attempting to live out their lives with some dignity and safety.

The CHAIRMAN. Thank you so much for your testimony. It is compelling. We are grateful you could be with us today, Mr. Clifford.

Senator Franken, if I could ask you to introduce our next witness.

STATEMENT OF HON. AL FRANKEN,
U.S. SENATOR FROM MINNESOTA

Senator FRANKEN. Thank you, Mr. Chairman.

It is my honor to introduce Chairman Darrell Seki of the Red Lake Band of Chippewa. Chairman Seki has served Red Lake in various roles over the past 40 years. He has served over a decade as treasurer of the Red Lake Tribal Council and last year, he was elected tribal chairman.

The Red Lake Band is far too familiar with tragedy. Just since March when Chairman Seki testified before a House committee on this very issue, Red Lake has lost two children to suicide.

Chairman Seki can speak not only to the challenge of addressing this immediate crisis but also to the struggle to fund services for Indian youth over the long term.

I am pleased to welcome you, Mr. Chairman, to the Indian Affairs Committee. I look forward to hearing your valuable perspective on how we can make a sustained effort to prevent suicide and how we can create a better future for our young people in Indian Country.

Thank you for being here.

STATEMENT OF HON. DARRELL G. SEKI, SR., CHAIRMAN, RED LAKE BAND OF CHIPPEWA INDIANS

Mr. SEKI. Thank you to Senator Franken for introducing me.

[Prayer in Native language.]

Mr. SEKI. Good afternoon, Chairman Barrasso, Vice Chairman Tester and members of the Committee.

Thank you for the opportunity to testify today about ending Native youth suicides. I will focus my testimony on youth suicide but I would also point out that Red Lake suffers from high suicide rates in people over 18 as well. Like our brothers and sisters at the Pine Ridge Reservation, the Red Lake Nation is experiencing high numbers of youth suicide, attempted suicide, suicide ideations and counseling referrals.

We are happy to hear Pine Ridge received a Department of Education SERV grant. Red Lake received a SERV grant and a SAMHSA grant 10 years ago after the Red Lake School shooting.

Operating these grant programs, we learned two big lessons. First, was that school counselors can make a huge difference, second, we learned programs like this only work if they can be financially sustained over many years. It is long, hard, slow work.

Just three months ago, we marked the 10-year anniversary of the Red Lake School shooting. Ten people lost their lives that day. Five were wounded and many other lives were changed forever. Although President George W. Bush promised we would not be forgotten, that promise has not endured.

Last year, Red Lake suffered four youth suicides, two girls and two boys. This year, we already have lost two more kids to suicide including a 9 year old boy just a few weeks ago.

Over the last year of school at Red Lake, there were more than 75 cases of suicide ideation. School wellness counselor intervention resulted in more than 40 students being placed under protective watch and sent to appropriate medical facilities for care.

The counselors initiated dozens of safety plans which drove us to get assistance when needed. This proves our counselors are doing their job. Counselors can and do save lives.

Because of staffing reductions and other sequestration, we are unable to reach all who need help. Anyone who thinks sequestration is not bad is dead wrong. Sequestration is a nightmare for tribes at Red Lake who must rely on Federal funding.

The current youth suicide intervention process usually ends without any continuing care. After the crisis is over, there are no financial resources for follow up treatment. That is like funding an emergency room with only hospital services for performing surgery without any post-op rehab services.

Students do not get needed after-care because of the Indian Health Service's staffing shortage. Often these shortages lead to wait times of several weeks for follow up care. This frustrates some families and they give up.

Last fall, my office conducted community meetings across our reservation focusing on suicide, drugs and bullying. In those meetings, we identified several obstacles to solving our suicide problem. Some of those obstacles include loss of our traditions in everyday life, lack of nearby facilities, needed after care services on reservations, more training in how to have difficult family conversations, and perhaps most important, parental drug use which includes alcohol. Our community members felt that solving drug abuse is critical in bringing an end to suicide.

The solutions we came up with can easily be summed up. We simply must restore our sense of community. We have a plan to end suicide on our reservation. Components of our plan include strengthening our wellness counselor program by doubling the number of counselors and social workers; improving the process for follow-up care; rebuilding hope by rebuilding our infrastructure; getting tough on drug offenders and precluding them from our land while building rehabilitative services for our members.

A key in building our rehabilitative services is the Tiwahe Initiative. We are very fortunate to have just been selected as one of the four tribes to participate in the pilot component of BIA's Tiwahe Initiative. The purpose of the Initiative is to address the underlying causes of poverty, domestic violence, substance abuse and suicide. Tiwahe utilizes integrated approaches to service delivery and redesign of the services offered by bringing all of our programs together.

We are going to break down the silos. We are going to find ways to implement what works. In building our infrastructure, we believe that hope is often fostered by prosperity. We have a plan to build our economy at Red Lake. We are focusing on our infrastructure like communications, roads, diversifying our tribal enterprises and improving local training programs in order to build our workforce.

Congress can help by ending sequestration for tribes. We will have more recurring dollars to support our efforts to end youth suicides. By supporting the Tiwahe Initiative, we can strengthen our social service and rehabilitation programs.

Congress needs to remove the obstacles imposed on tribes through a process of short term grants. Summed up, our big message is that only sustained funding of affected programs will end youth suicides in Indian Country. Red Lake has a plan to do that but we need sustained funding to do so.

I want to thank the Committee for giving me this opportunity to speak on behalf of Red Lake Nation.

[The prepared statement of Mr. Seki follows:]

PREPARED STATEMENT OF HON. DARRELL G. SEKI SR., CHAIRMAN, RED LAKE BAND OF CHIPPEWA INDIANS

Mr. Chairman, I thank you and the other distinguished members of the Committee for this opportunity to provide testimony on behalf of the Red Lake Band of Chippewa Indians, and for your attention on the problem of native youth suicides. For statistical purposes I will focus my testimony on youth under 18, but I would also point out Red Lake suffers from high suicide rates in over 18 years as well.

On behalf of the Red Lake Nation, I want to extend my sympathies to my brother Mr. Yellow Bird Steele, and the people of Pine Ridge. The Red Lake Nation is also experiencing high numbers of youth suicides, attempted suicides, suicide ideations, and counselling referrals. We are happy you received a Department of Education SERV grant. Red Lake received a SERV grant and a SAMHSA grant 10 years ago after the Red Lake School Shooting. Two lessons we learned are that school counsellors can make a huge difference and programs like this only work if they can be financially sustained over time.

About Red Lake Band of Chippewa Indians

Red Lake is a fairly large tribe with 12,000 members. Our 840,000 acre reservation is held in trust for the tribe by the United States. While it has been diminished in size, our reservation has never been broken apart or allotted to individuals. Nor has it been subjected to the criminal or civil jurisdiction of the State of Minnesota. Thus, we have a large land area over which we exercise full governmental authority and control, in conjunction with the United States. At the same time, due in part to our remote location, we have few jobs available on our reservation. While the unemployment rate in Minnesota is 3.7 percent, ours remains at an outrageously high level of about 50 percent. The lack of infrastructure such as good roads, communications, technology and other necessary infrastructure continues to hold back economic development and job opportunities.

Red Lake Suicide Rates and Intervention Process

Health information laws constrain our ability to consolidate suicide data. The School district, law enforcement and our health services all collect data in different ways, which makes analysis of suicide-related data difficult. Focusing on just health services, the data shows that last year we had four youth suicides-two girls and two boys-and there were 63 cases of suicide ideation. Due to Wellness Counselor interventions, 34 students were placed under protective watch and sent to appropriate medical facilities for care. The counselors initiated dozens of Safety Plans with students to get assistance when needed. This proves the counselors are doing their job, and they can and do save lives. But because of staffing reductions under sequestration, we are unable to reach all who need help. Anyone who thinks sequestration is not so bad is dead wrong. Sequestration is a nightmare for tribes who must rely on federal funding.

The current youth suicide intervention process ultimately ends with no lasting service. For example, when a student is having a problem in our school, the teacher will contact of a wellness counselor. The wellness counselor will first talk with the child and then take the child to the school social worker. If the child meets all the signs of suicidal behavior the child is taken to the hospital emergency room. After a doctor evaluates the child the hospital mental health staff will further evaluate to determine whether the child should go to a special facility for further treatment and observation. In this example, the child visited four separately funded programs, the independent school district, Red Lake Comprehensive Health Services, Indian Health Services—Emergency and Indian Health Services—Behavioral Health and if they are forwarded to another facility, it represents yet another funding source. At Red Lake, because of staffing shortages, it is well documented that Indian Health Service follow up care is always backed up by several weeks and children must wait weeks in order to be seen for follow up.

The History of Our Suicide Problem

Last fall, my office conducted community meetings focusing on suicide, drugs and bullying. We visited all four of our tribal communities and had great attendance and participation from our members. From our community meetings our members identified several long-standing obstacles to solving our social ills including youth suicide. Some of those obstacles include: loss of our traditions in everyday life; lack of facilities nearby; no aftercare in our land; inability to have "difficult" conversations; and perhaps most importantly, parental drug use-which includes alcohol. Our community members felt that solving drug abuse and bullying are critical needs in bringing about an end to suicide. The solutions our community came up with can easily be summed up; restore our sense of community.

The trail to suicide isn't far from lack of job opportunities. A lack of employment opportunities results in poverty and disparity. Poverty and disparity can lead to drugs and addiction. Drug addiction leads to the tear down of our families, which often precipitates high suicide rates.

But drugs are not the only source of our high suicide rate. Just three months ago, we marked the 10th anniversary of the Red Lake School shooting. 10 people lost their lives that day, 5 were wounded, and many other lives were changed forever. Today, a lot of those people are still suffering from the horror they faced that day. The story gets even more tragic when we consider that President George W. Bush told Red Lake the Government would come to our aid, and we would not be forgotten. But that promise did not endure.

I talked about Red Lake's youth suicide problem at the House Interior Appropriations Committee last March. Since that time two more kids committed suicide, including a nine year old boy just three weeks ago. I pointed out during the March hearing that for three years now, sequestration took about $1.5 million each year from Red Lake's BIA and IHS base programs, and additional amounts from formula-based programs. This has made it very difficult for us to provide any sustained assistance to combat youth suicide. Grants are very difficult to apply for and to manage, and they don't last. Sustained funding is our only hope to make a difference.

How Red Lake Can End Suicide on Our Reservation

a. Expanding our Wellness Counselor Program

Our Tribal Health program funds the Red Lake Schools' Wellness Program, which provides counselors to help students when they have problems and are thinking of harming themselves. It began after the School shooting, with help from a SAMHSA grant. The grant ended two years later, so the Tribe has had to pick up the tab ever since. Because of sequestration we had to cut the number of wellness counselors from 8 to 5, which is not nearly enough to assist hundreds of students in four schools. Additionally, we have only two school social workers, they are the specialists who usually make the first diagnosis of a problem. The wellness counselors and social workers in our schools are the critical front-line components of our suicide prevention plan. We need to at least double their numbers this year: from 5 to 10 wellness counselors; and from 2 to 4 social workers.

b. Attacking Our Drug Problem

Drugs are a major factor in our suicide rates and we have taken a hard line against offenders. Within the last few weeks federal agents and our tribal police force arrested 41 people involved in trafficking drugs. The traffickers moved drugs such as heroin, methamphetamine and prescription pills in to Red Lake. We continue to work with our law enforcement partners and the United States Attorney's Office to expand on the number of drug busts. And that isn't all, the Red Lake Band of Chippewa Indians has also permanently removed many non-member drug Dealers from our lands.

c. Large Concentrated Multi-Prong Push

The Band will take a multi-program rehabilitative approach to address suicide and the underlying causes we see in Red Lake. We are very fortunate to have just been selected as one of four tribes to participate in the BIA's Tiwahe Initiative. The purpose of the Tiwahe Initiative is to address the underlying causes of poverty, domestic violence, substance abuse, and suicide, by utilizing an integrated approach to service delivery, and redesign of the services offered. We are bringing all of our programs together, we are going to break down the silos, and we are going to find out what works and does not work, and we're going to find a way to implement what works. We recently formed a suicide prevention task force to better coordinate mental health and suicide prevention services.

d. Building Infrastructure

Hope is often fostered by prosperity. Providing adequate funding for governmental functions allows us to spend what little of our own money we have on economic development. We have a plan to build our economy in Red Lake. We are focusing on things that never leave the reservation; our infrastructure like communications and roads, and improving local training programs in order to build our workforce.

How Congress Can Help Red Lake to Accomplish Our Plan

Congress can help tribes reduce suicide by ending sequestration and by finding a way to provide additional and sustained funding. Red Lake, like many government agencies, suffers from compartmentalization of many services, including for mental health and suicide prevention. This makes it difficult to coordinate an effective approach to combatting the problem. And it makes it difficult for community members to know what services are available and where to go for help. Compartmentalization is partly the result of the fact that most funding to address mental health comes in the form of grants. Silos are created because granting agencies have their own unique funding requirements, and they award funds to different types of grantees (e.g. Department of Education to schools; HHS to health centers; DOJ and SAMHSA to tribal governments).

I have already alluded to it, but one thing we know about Indian Country is that grants often do not work. Grants are short term and often non-strategic. Further, federal application and reporting requirements are cumbersome and require significant resources to complete. Our SAMHSA grant was helpful but it only lasted two years.

The problem with grants is an issue that national scholars have noted. Miriam Jorgensen, the editor of ''Rebuilding Native Nations'' noted that often, Indian Tribes are unable to set their own development agenda—they must pattern it to obtain grants. Further Ms. Jorgensen pointed out, ''few dollars come to Native Nations via block grants, a mechanism that would place more decisionmaking power in Indians hands.''

Compounding the problems associated with grants, the only recurring funding we could count on, from BIA and IHS, has been hammered by sequestration and at least 14 different across the board rescissions. Congress could aid in reducing our suicide rate by ending sequestration in Indian Country, and returning our sequestered funds to us.

In summary, in order to end suicide in Red Lake we need to better understand what we are doing right, and what we are doing wrong. We are optimistic that Red Lake's participation in the Tiwahe Initiative will serve as the springboard to make changes that will work. Poverty brings about hopelessness and despair. Drugs that follow poverty have destroyed our understanding of family. The horrors of the school shooting still linger, and there is also generational trauma. Our community members feel we need to restore our sense of community. Sequestration has limited our ability to address our problems. Grants are not the answer-they set programs up for failure. Only sustained funding of effective programs will end youth suicides in Indian Country. Red Lake has a plan to do that, but we need sustained funding to do so.

Thank you for allowing me to provide testimony today on the important topic of ending Native Youth Suicides.

The CHAIRMAN. Thank you very much, Chairman Seki.
Dr. LaFromboise.

STATEMENT OF TERESA D. LAFROMBOISE, Ph.D., PROFESSOR, DEVELOPMENTAL AND PSYCHOLOGICAL SCIENCES, GRADUATE SCHOOL OF EDUCATION, STANFORD UNIVERSITY

Dr. LaFROMBOISE. Good afternoon, Mr. Chairman and members of the Committee. I am grateful for the opportunity to present testimony on a topic of urgent importance in Indian Country.

I have been working in the field over American Indian suicide prevention since 1989. I began at the invitation of Mr. Hayes Lewis, the Superintendent of the Zuni Public School District. He made a request to me at Stanford to bring a team of educators and health promotion specialists from Stanford University to the Pueblo of Zuni to help community experts develop a culturally grounded youth suicide prevention intervention.

Over the course of three years, our team worked in Zuni to develop a life skills curriculum, to consult with the Zuni Board of Education and the Zuni Tribal Council, and conduct an outcome study of the curriculum we developed. We compared students in the curriculum with those who were not. We found those in the curriculum, the Zuni Life Skills Curriculum, displayed less suicidal ideation, suicide attempts, less hopelessness, greater self-efficacy to manage anger, and greater effectiveness in helping a suicidal friend solve problems and to go to someone for help.

Today, I would like to talk a little bit about the derivative of the Zuni Life Skills which is the American Indian Life Skills. I would also like to talk about four other evidence-based interventions used in Indian communities and found to be effective in reducing suicide. The evaluations were not with Native communities but with communities across mainstream society. I think that might provide some help.

When Mr. Lewis invited us to develop this curriculum, we were invited only to do work with the Zuni high school. We did not have a lot of experience, although I did teach junior high and high school, so I learned a lot about school-based suicide prevention.

The rationale for suicide prevention in schools hinges on the recognition that a significant amount of suicidal behavior occurs among ostensibly well-functioning students. The idea is to do a population-based strategy of exposing all students to suicide awareness and skills about suicide so that it can reach the greatest number of students who will then help the smaller number of students who are at risk.

These programs primarily target an individual student's thinking and behavior. The ultimate goal is to help at-risk students receive psychological treatment before they become acutely suicidal. The type of approaches then in schools for suicide prevention consists of awareness and education curricula, peer leadership training, skills training, gatekeeper training and screening.

The Zuni Life Skills was expanded to have examples from a number of different tribes so that we could reach a more diverse group of people. The emphasis is social skills training and intervention that emphasizes the fact that suicide is an action and a behavior rather than focusing on it as a mental illness.

This curriculum has seven major themes: building self-esteem; identifying emotions and stress; increasing communication and problem-solving skills; recognizing self-destructive behavior and finding ways to eliminate it; learning information about suicide; helping a suicidal friend go for help; and planning ahead for a great future.

You may say, what is cultural about that? There are a number of opportunities for cultural considerations in this curriculum but more of the scenarios in it emphasize realistic situations that occur in Native communities. We talk about culturally appropriate ways to express emotions and grief.

Tribal community members are encouraged to be the ones that deliver the intervention. Tribal community members are invited into a number of the sessions to share cultural teachings and to model cultural coping perspectives. It is cultural. This has been offered in a number of schools but it is also offered in cultural camps, local recreation and sports programs, Boys and Girls Clubs, Upward Bound, treatment centers, tribal colleges and tribal youth employment.

It has been adapted in recent years for urban and suburban settings and in some tribal communities, a few, such as the Spirit Lake Dakota Tribe which has adapted it for their local community values and norms.

I have had the opportunity of training community members from over 100 reservations that have participated in these trainings. Now we are working on internet applications in order to provide technical assistance after these trainings.

I want to talk about four other programs. Basically, the reason I selected these four is that they have a history of implementation in Indian communities and also have yielded outcomes in randomized controlled trials.

The first one is Sources of Strength. This was a program developed out of the United Tribes in Bismarck and later adapted for mainstream society. Basically, the emphasis of this program is a lot of positive messaging, suicidal awareness and training of peer leaders, the idea being that once the students identify who are the adults in the school who are really supportive of them as mentors and the peer leaders, those at risk might go to these peer leaders to get help. At three month follow-up, participants in Sources of Strength reported reduced suicide attempts and increased knowledge about suicide.

Another program is called Reconnecting Youth. I learned about that because I was looking for a comparative treatment to evaluate the American Indian Life Skills. This was already being used at a number of reservations.

The emphasis on this one is to work with at-risk students to help them be able to monitor their own substance use and monitor their attendance in school. This is like the last stop before getting kicked out of school. In this program, basically they learn rather than be kicked out for being out of control, or poor attendance or coming to school loaded, they learn how to manage this.

I have to say we used this with middle school students. Over only 10 months, we saw reduced hopelessness at post-test and reduced suicidal ideation. Then at one year follow-up, we saw even greater gains.

Another one is a shorter version of this called CAST, made by the same developers. Basically, it is a shortened version of Reconnecting Youth.

Finally, I want to talk about the Good Behavior Game. I found out about these when I served on the National Academy of Sciences and Institutes of Medicine's task force which developed a book, all this is outlined in there, to prevent behavioral, emotional and mental disorders in young children.

The Good Behavior Game has been touted as the most effective behavioral vaccine. This is actually not a program; it is a strategy where in working with elementary children, they learn self-regulation. The teacher basically divides the class into teams. Teams are reinforced for staying on task, doing the appropriate thing, not talking out of turn, and focusing on what they are doing for a while.

I know it sounds manipulative. What they are learning is self-regulation. I have to say this has been used with First Nations elementary children and Metis Children in Canada.

The important results of this is that following these elementary school children into adolescence, they were just exposed to it in elementary, and by adolescence they had less impulsive, disruptive behavior, less substance use, drug addiction, lower rates of suicidal ideation and suicidal attempts. That is quite a nice long term effect.

The CHAIRMAN. Doctor, if you have any last summation you want to make, because I know there are a number of questions.

Dr. LaFROMBOISE. I am so sorry.

Basically, I think I would concur in what people have indicated as solutions to this. Unfortunately, what we have here is a situation where we do not have enough psychologists or behavioral health specialists to meet the need.

In schools, it is very difficult to implement because administrators are very concerned about making grade in terms of AYP and high stakes testing. It is very difficult.

I am suggesting that we really turn to looking at Masters level people. We have more jobs for Masters level people that will supplement the already existing counseling staff in schools and help with this kind of work because you can see the results. They can work. We just need the staff in order to deliver it.

Thank you.

[The prepared statement of Ms. LaFromboise follows:]

PREPARED STATEMENT OF TERESA D. LAFROMBOISE, PH.D., PROFESSOR, DEVELOPMENTAL AND PSYCHOLOGICAL SCIENCES, GRADUATE SCHOOL OF EDUCATION, STANFORD UNIVERSITY

Good afternoon Mr. Chairman and members of the committee. I am grateful for the opportunity to present testimony on a topic of urgent importance in Indian Country, that is, the need for effective interventions to reduce the exceedingly high rates of Native American youth suicide.

My name is Teresa LaFromboise. I am a Professor of Psychological and Developmental Sciences at the Graduate School of Education at Stanford University. I have been working in the field of American Indian/Alaska Native (AI/AN) youth suicide prevention since 1989.

The work began in response to a request from Mr. Hayes Lewis, the Superintendent of the Zuni Public School District, that I bring a team of educators and health promotion specialists from Stanford University to the Pueblo of Zuni to help community experts develop a culturally-grounded youth suicide prevention intervention.

Over the course of three years we worked in Zuni to develop life skills pedagogy and curriculum lessons, consult with the Zuni Board of Education and the Zuni Tribal Council, and conduct an outcome study to assess the psychological impact of the curriculum (LaFromboise & Lewis, 2008) . This outcome evaluation demonstrated the following effects: less suicidal ideation and suicide attempts, less hopelessness, greater self-efficacy to manage anger, and greater effectiveness in helping a suicidal friend solve problems and go for help among participants in the Zuni Life Skills treatment group as compared to those in the no-treatment comparison group (LaFromboise & Howard-Pitney, 1995).

Today, I want to provide a brief overview of ongoing work associated with American Indian Life Skills (AILS) and introduce four other evidence-based interventions delivered in school settings that have produced favorable outcomes in youth suicide prevention. I will discuss some of the limitations of interventions that focus solely on psychological rather than social, cultural and spiritual issues that may be more relevant in Native American youth suicide prevention. Finally, I will offer some recommendations concerning how we might more effectively reverse the rates of youth suicide within tribal communities.

Promising Practices in School Based Suicide Prevention

When we were invited to develop an intervention in Zuni we were only allowed access to the Zuni High School. Thus we learned a lot about suicide prevention in schools. The rationale for schools adopting suicide prevention programs hinges upon recognition that a significant amount of suicidal behavior occurs among ostensibly, well-functioning students. School suicide prevention programs try to reach the greatest number of students through population-based strategies to identify and assist the smaller number of students who are at risk. They primarily target an individual student's thinking and behavior. The ultimate goal is to help at-risk students receive psychological treatment before they become acutely suicidal.

Presently, there are five main types of suicide prevention interventions in schools: (a) awareness/education curricula, (b) peer leadership training, (c) skills training, (d) gatekeeper training and (e) screening. *Awareness/education curricula* focuses on increasing accurate knowledge about suicide, and encourages self-disclosure among peers to develop positive attitudes toward seeking help. *Peer leadership* training assists student leaders in learning to respond to suicidal peers and then to refer them to a "trusted adult" for further referral to treatment. *Skills training* fosters the growth of skills to support protective factors in the prevention of suicide (e.g., problem solving, self-regulation). Emphasis is also placed on the reduction of risk factors to prevent the development of suicidal behavior (e.g., depression, substance abuse, anger regulation). *Gatekeeper training* teaches school staff, students and their parents about symptoms of suicide, and additionally provides information regarding risk and protective factors in order to improve identification and referral of at-risk students to available resources. Lastly, *screening* programs assess suicidal ideation, depression symptoms, and other clinical mental health disorders (including multiple problems such as depression along with disturbed eating or binge drinking) in order to refer students displaying disorder to psychological services.

American Indian Life Skills

The success of the Zuni Life Skills Development Curriculum bolstered a more Native American generic version entitled the *American Indian Life Skills Development Curriculum* (AILS) which is available to any tribe or community that is searching for adolescent suicide prevention and life empowerment programs (LaFromboise, 1996).

AILS is a universal, community-driven suicide prevention intervention emphasizing social cognitive skills training to reduce suicidal behaviors . AILS strongly emphasizes suicide as an action and behavior rather than the result of mental illness. It emphasizes an array of psychosocial skills necessary for effectively dealing with everyday life such as: emotional regulation, mindfulness, problem solving, and anger regulation. It focuses on 7 main themes: (1) building self-esteem; (2) identifying emotions and stress; (3) increasing communication and problem-solving skills; (4) recognizing self-destructive behavior and finding ways to eliminate it; (5) learning information about suicide; (6) helping a suicidal friend go for help, and (7) planning ahead for a great future.

A number of cultural considerations were considered in the design of this intervention. The curriculum is full of realistic situations that occur in AI/AN communities and homes. Lessons in AILS encourages culturally appropriate ways that students can express emotions like grief or anger. The preferred interventionist of AILS is a professionally trained community member. Additional community members are invited into AILS sessions at relevant times to share cultural teachings and model cultural coping perspectives.

Ideally, AILS is offered in a required course such and social studies or language arts. However, AILS has been taught in culture camps, local recreation and sports camps, tribal youth employment and training programs, Upward Bound, treatment centers, and tribal colleges. It has been adapted for AI/AN adolescents in urban and suburban settings. In addition, tribal communities such as the Spirit Lake Dakota tribe have adapted AILS to their local community values and norms.

Community members, teachers and behavioral health specialists from over 100 reservations have participated in AILS trainings. Currently, we are working on Internet applications for providing on-going technical assistance to those who are implementing AILS following an initial 3-day Key Leader Orientation training.

Schools as Sites for Suicide Prevention

From my experience in this field and from systematic review of research on school-based suicide prevention programs, I have found a growing number of potentially effective mainstream programs that could be of help in reducing Native American youth suicide. I selected the following evidence-based programs to highlight today because they each have some history of implementation in AI/AN communities and they have been found to yield outcomes associated with the prevention of adolescent suicide with diverse populations (LaFromboise & Hussain, in press).

Sources of Strength (SOS). SOS is a universal program (meaning that it is offered to all students in a school) that emphasizes awareness/education and peer leadership to reduce suicidal behaviors (LoMurray, 2005). Its curriculum includes suicide awareness, positive messaging, empowering activities and screening strategies. Peer leaders are trained in responding to students who display risk factors for suicide, directing them to a trusted adult for further support. Originally designed for youth living in rural areas near United Tribes in Bismarck, North Dakota to tackle issues related to suicide, such as violence and substance use, SOS was later modified for widespread use with students from diverse backgrounds across the United States. At a 3-month follow up, participants in SOS reported reduced suicide attempts and increased knowledge about suicide (Aseltine, James, Schilling, & Glanovsky, 2007).

Reconnecting Youth (RY). RY is a selected intervention utilizing a life-skills training approach which targets high school students who demonstrate poor academic achievement, are at risk for dropping out of school and exhibit maladaptive symptoms like aggressive behavior (Eggert & Nicholas, 2004). RY emphasizes the prevention of substance use and emotional distress while fostering resilience. Opportunity for social bonding is also achieved through intervention activities which form connections within the school and encourage parent involvement. Native American RY participants have reported reduced hopelessness and suicidal ideation immediately following the intervention and at 1-year follow up (LaFromboise & Malik, 2012).

Coping and Support Training (CAST). CAST is a selected prevention program adapted from RY that uses a skills-training approach with high school students following their referral to the program based upon initial screening. CAST consists of 12 sessions given over 6 weeks administered by service providers (e.g., teachers, nurses). CAST focuses on mood management and school performance and emphasizes decreased involvement with illicit substances. Participants of CAST have demonstrated increased problem solving skills, perceived family support and self-control, and decreased symptoms of depression and hopelessness (Thompson, Eggert, Randell & Pike, 2001).

Good Behavior Game (GBG). GBG is a behavior management approach that has evolved into a universal, primary prevention program for elementary school students to teach self-regulation skills (Barrish, Saunders, & Wolf, 1969). The GBG socializes children into displaying cooperative rather than disruptive or aggressive behavior, both of which are risk factors for substance abuse and suicide. To play the GBG a teacher splits the classroom into two or more teams which are rewarded for being adaptive to academic social expectations (e.g., being on task for brief periods of time, not talking out of turn). Eventually they are expected to be cooperative for longer periods of time. The winner of the GBG is the team with the least amount of infractions.

GBG has demonstrated long-term effects (following elementary school-age participants on into adolescence) on decreased impulsive/disruptive behavior, substance use, drug addictions, and lower rates of suicidal ideation and suicide attempts (Kellam et al., 2008). By incorporating the program into the classroom at an early age, there is a high cost-effectiveness ratio.

Lessons Learned

From having either carefully reviewed, implemented or tested each these programs, I found that it is very difficult to influence schools to engage in primary prevention. "School administrators and teachers working in public schools serving Indian populations are so bent upon meeting the high stakes demands of testing and Adequate Yearly Progress (AYP) that they have no time to do more than the minimum expected when it comes to responding to the emotional and cultural needs of Native American students" (Testimony of Hayes A. Lewis, Youth Suicide in Indian Country, February 26, 2009, p.4). It takes advocacy from community champions (e.g., tribal council members, members of prevention committees and parents) to influence school administrators to adopt programs sensitive to the social emotional needs of youth.

Most of these interventions rely on the referral of at-risk students to psychological treatment before they become acutely suicidal. However, many rural AI/AN communities have limited school counseling services or behavioral health services. When formal mental health services are staffed by AI/AN behavioral health specialists those services are in high demand. When they are staffed by service providers from outside the community they may be underutilized due to the stigma of seeking help from those who seemingly represent the group that marginalizes and oppresses them. The ultimate effectiveness of the prevention program, to save lives, relies on youth initiating or completing care.

I also found that most individually focused "off the shelf interventions" do not address key perceived contributions to AI/AN suicide such as historical oppression, intergenerational trauma, prejudice and discrimination and other forms of collective disempowerment. Thus the protocols upon which these interventions were tested are either short lived or, in the best case scenario, modified to address more relevant social justice issues in Indian Country.

Finally, those AI/AN communities, who actually implement programs such as the ones I have just reviewed and who find them intuitively "helpful," are often reluctant to engage in further assessment of their effectiveness within their own community. I believe that this type of assessment would be helpful in guiding decisions about modifications to the intervention to better meet local community needs and norms or concerning whether or not to continue efforts toward sustaining the intervention overtime.

Recommendations

I respectfully offer the following recommendations to strengthen tribal capacity to improve service delivery to prevent Native youth suicide based upon my observations, research, and training experiences.

Expand the number of empirically-validated suicide prevention interventions and evaluate their adaptation and implementation in diverse AI/AN contexts.

School-based suicide prevention programs began in 1984 in reaction to a significant escalating trend in suicidal behavior among adolescents in many Western industrialized countries. Considering the relatively new introduction of prevention intervention to this complicated problem, issues with customized delivery that target specific variables such as ethnic/racial group background, cultural involvement, and tribal diversity still need significant innovation and evaluation.

Make a commitment to continue to support the dissemination of valued community-driven approaches to suicide prevention across Indian Country.

There is a sense of urgency among tribal leaders to preserve cultural ways of knowing before the knowledge keepers are gone. Research indicates that communities with higher levels of political and cultural engagement have lower suicide rates. Certain individual protective factors for Native youth suicide prevention include cultural identity and engagement in cultural activities as well as school completion. This presents a window of opportunity for collaboration between community leaders and prevention scientists to develop services that reflect community priorities and practices and to mobilize available support systems to prevent suicide.

Encourage and support research on the interaction of community-level processes, family systems, and individual psychology that affect the well-being and resilience of Native youth.

Historically suicide prevention has focused on the treatment of the individual and that type of intervention should continue but not at the cost of ignoring the gestalt of the disorder. Specific efforts have evolved for the last decades or two on economically viable, rapidly deployed and clinically efficacious efforts to target not only the individual but the larger system- from social media to society and everything in between. Let us continue that momentum.

Tribal communities have practiced "integrated care" among individuals and families for generations but usually without adequate resources. Let us support continuation of those cultural practices and healing traditions.

Thank you for providing this opportunity.

References

Barrish, H.H., Saunders, M., & Wolf, M.M. (1969). Good Behavior Game: Effects of individual contingencies for group consequences on disruptive behavior in a classroom. *Journal of Applied Behavior Analysis, 2,* 119–124. Retrieved from *http://search.proquest.com/docview/615628148?accountid=14026*

Eggert, L.L., & Nicholas, L. J. (2004). *Reconnecting youth.* Bloomington, IN: National Educational Service.

Kellam, S.G., Brown, H.C., Poduska, J.M., Ialongo, N.S., Wang, W., Toyinbo, P., & Wilcox, H.C. (2008). Effects of a universal classroom behavior management program in first and second grades on young adult behavioral, psychiatric, and social outcomes. *Drug and Alcohol Dependence, 95,* S5–S28. doi: 10.1016/j.drugalcdep.2008.01.004

LaFromboise, T.D. (1996). *American Indian Life Skills Development Curriculum.* Madison, WI: University of Wisconsin Press.

47

LaFromboise, T.D., & Howard-Pitney, B. (1995). The Zuni Life Skills Development Curriculum: Description and evaluation of a suicide prevention program. *Journal of Counseling Psychology,* 42, 479–486. doi: 10.1037/0022–0167.42.4.47

LaFromboise, T.D., & Hussain, S. (in press). School-based adolescent suicide prevention. In L. Bosworth (Eds.). *Prevention Science in School Settings: Complex Relationships and Processes.* New York: Springer.

LaFromboise, T.D., & Lewis, H.A. (2008). The Zuni Life Skills Development Program: A school/community-based suicide prevention intervention. *Suicide and Life-Threatening Behavior,* 38, 343–353. doi: 10.1521/suli.2008.38.3.343

LaFromboise, T.D., & Malik, S.S. (2012, May). *Development of the American Indian Life Skills Curriculum: Middle School Version.* Poster presentation, Second Biennial Conference of the Society for the Psychological Study of Ethnic Minority Issues. Ann Arbor, MI.

LoMurray, M. (2005). *Sources of Strength facilitators guide: Suicide prevention peer gatekeeper training.* Bismarck, ND: The North Dakota Suicide Prevention Project.

Thompson, E. A., Eggert, L. L., Randell, B. P., & Pike, K. C. (2001). Evaluation of indicated suicide risk prevention approaches for potential high school dropouts. *American Journal of Public Health,* 91, 742–752. doi: 0.2105/AJPH.91.5.742

Wexler, L., Chandler, M., Gone, J., Cwik, M., Kirmayer, L., LaFromboise, T., Brockie, T., O'Keefe, V., Walkup, J., & Allen, J. (2015). Advancing suicide prevention research with rural American Indian and Alaska Native populations. *American Journal of Public Health.*

The CHAIRMAN. Thank you so very much.

I want to thank all of our witnesses for their testimony.

I will now turn to questions from the Committee, starting with Senator Tester.

Senator TESTER. Thank you, Mr. Chairman.

I want to go back to you, Teresa. Your Ph.D is in what?

Dr. LaFROMBOISE. Counseling Psychology.

Senator TESTER. I would ask you to be as concise as you possibly can.

Senator Udall went down the litany of things faced in Indian Country in his opening statement: alcohol, drug abuse, physical abuse, poor nutrition, poor schools, domestic violence, poverty, and overcrowded housing. You know the statistics probably better than anyone up here. The rate at which Native Americans commit suicide is the highest of any minority in the Country. In 15 to 34 year olds, the rate is twice that of anybody else.

What do we do about this? If there is alcohol abuse, drug abuse by parents or the potential person who is going to commit suicide, combine that with poor nutrition and poor schools, where do you start?

Dr. LaFROMBOISE. First, I understand what you are alluding to. You are alluding to all these intense social determinants of behavior. Probably you are thinking I am naive to focus on the individual.

Senator TESTER. No, no. I want to do to solve the problem.

Dr. LaFROMBOISE. Here is what I would suggest. All these problems need to be solved. One thing we do know about the resilience literature is that the children who are resilient, meaning they are able to thrive in spite of all this adversity, are children who are able to manage their emotions and are able to stay detached from situations and are able to have a strong identity.

All these things these kinds of program do. They emphasize the protective factors.

Senator TESTER. The resilience is taught where, in school?

Dr. LAFROMBOISE. Resilience begins as a child.

Senator TESTER. I know, but when you have dysfunction, alcoholism, and housing problems, where the hell are they going to learn resilience?

Dr. LAFROMBOISE. They can begin to learn it in school. Obviously I am an educator, so I think of school. The schools are sanctuaries. For some children, this is the only place they get a meal. For some, this is the only place they feel safe.

That is why I am thinking of this arena as the place where we can really marshal some forces to try to help them. There are some wonderful programs. I remember Duane Mackey had a program a number of years ago called The Heart Room. This heart room was in schools.

Children went into the heart room on Friday for prayer and meditation and to prepare for what they were going to have to go through over the weekend. They came back into that heart room on Monday in order to decompress and be ready to focus in school.

Obviously, we need so much more. It would be nice if we could do this kind of work in families. Unfortunately, we really did not have access to families.

Senator TESTER. Thank you.

A month or two months ago, we had a hearing here on schools about being subpar, cold, lack of academic materials, and the lack of good teachers. We have a lot of problems.

I want to go over to Mr. McSwain. It is a fact and folks have testified here today about recruitment and retention of dedicated, high quality health care providers as critical for your work at IHS. You indicated four different scholarship and loan repayment programs to recruit health care professionals in the IHS service areas.

It is known, it is not a secret, that there is a shortage of IHS mental health providers. Why has IHS never employed the Indian Health Service Mental Health Prevention and Treatment Loan Repayment Program?

Mr. MCSWAIN. Senator, that is a good question.

I know we have been working on our own loan repayment, our own scholarship program and we have been using the National Health Service Corps Loan Repayment Program and using their scholars but we have not gone beyond that.

Senator TESTER. To me, it sounds like the perfect program to try to get folks into Indian Country who can help. The professor talked about more professionals in Indian Country can help. Are there any plans to enact it? Do you have the dough to do it? What is the problem?

Mr. MCSWAIN. A good point, because we just recently were identifying some vacancies but it was a matter of getting the people there in these remote locations. That is a challenge. I think Councilman Clifford mentioned that one of the biggest barriers to getting people out there is housing.

Senator TESTER. Yes, but you also have to enact that program. I was going to ask you the same question I asked the Professor. What are some of the programs that work for youth? I cannot because I have run out of time.

I want to say thank you guys very much for your testimony. We have to deal with this issue. If we do not deal with this issue, it is not going to go away; it is not going to get better. It is going to be here and it is going to get worse.

Whether it is working with the Administration or with individual tribes in Indian Country, we have to deal with this.

I appreciate you guys making the trek to Washington, D.C. Once again, this is the start of another conversation that I hope ends up in something that will functionally fix the problem.

The CHAIRMAN. Thank you, Senator Tester.

Senator Daines?

STATEMENT OF HON. STEVE DAINES, U.S. SENATOR FROM MONTANA

Senator DAINES. Thank you, Senator Tester, for that.

We both represent the State of Montana. I was meeting with four Montanans who came to my office yesterday. Montana has the highest per capita suicide rates in the Nation. We are number one.

It is a combination of a lot of factors. Certainly we have a high Native population. We talked about that here today. We have a high per capita veteran population. There is a crisis in our home State.

Mr. Chairman, thank you for holding this hearing. It is a tough topic to talk about but one we cannot ignore.

Dr. LaFromboise, you mentioned the need for the culturally-based suicide prevention programs. I was struck with your academic biography as a professor at Stanford and working in American Indian and Alaska Native youth suicide prevention since 1989, for more than 25 years, so we are glad to have your expertise.

I want to thank all of you for your testimonies today. I wish there was more time.

One of my constituents, Dustin Monroe, is the head of a group called Native Generational Change in Montana. He is an Assiniboine Black Feet tribal member, an Iraq veteran of the 25th Infantry Division. He is working on preventing youth suicide among Natives in rural communities.

One of the problems he has brought up is the lack of programs that adequately address the cultural differences that might exist between Indians and non-Indians with regard to suicide prevention and counseling. For example, Dustin mentions talking about the deceased might be therapeutic to some, but it could be very troubling to a Native population.

How well do you believe our suicide prevention or counseling programs take these cultural differences into account?

Dr. LAFROMBOISE. Certainly, the American Indian Life Skills has, because at the very beginning, the emphasis is saying that people who are doing this know best their own cultural teachings and that they should be respected. Therefore, they would be the ones to filter the information.

We do not encourage people to think about the deceased. We do have one lesson on grief because we feel that people need to think about stages of grief.

You are absolutely right. We do know from our research that people who have a strong cultural identity and strong involvement in cultural practices are certainly less likely to be involved in suicide. We also know that communities that have strong political engagement are in charge of most of what is going on in their community and strong practices.

I am not saying these things should be replaced. One of my recommendations would be that we should also increase the resources to help support community-driven interventions much like the individual you are talking about. I do not think one should replace the other. That is why I think it kind of helps to keep one in school and the other in the community because we are not interfering with each other.

Senator DAINES. Thank you.

You mentioned expanding the number of empirically-driven suicide interventions for school-based programs. I was struck by your comments to Senator Tester about how the school, for some young people, is the safe place they can go during the day and the week.

Given the limited dollars we have for all these programs. Where you look at empirically-based, outcome-based metrics, what programs are working, what programs are not working? In the zero sum game we face often here in Washington, D.C., what programs should we stop and double down on other programs that are working? What is not working and what is working?

Dr. LAFROMBOISE. I think it is very important to have gatekeeper training but I think the research would say that it does not really impact people as much as we think it does but it does help individuals who have already gone through the process of asking someone if they are suicidal and helps strengthen their skills.

For individuals that have never asked the question, they can go through gatekeeper training and come out and still never ask the question. That is one a lot of money is appropriated for but I am not really sure how well that works.

Senator DAINES. Before I run out of time, I want to ask Councilman Clifford from Pine Ridge a question.

Yesterday's conversation revolved around having a job, how that was a place to go, to work and when you are in poverty, the statistics you shared from Pine Ridge are staggering. What role does having a job and having employment play in trying to reduce suicide?

Mr. CLIFFORD. It gives a person something to do and also to look forward to a paycheck and paying their bills and being able to assist. I like your conversation about the cultural elements and the academic part. I think that has a lot to do with it and ties into being a working person. The cultural relevance of it is being able to share with what we grew up with and actually knowing.

The comparison and the so-called scientifically proven evidence, the cultural relevancy you cannot scientifically put a number on it. We know it works and it is there. It has always worked for many years.

I am reminded of the coffee shop story of a young lady in school and having a job. Not long ago, this young lady was feeling bad, suicidal tendencies and the ideations that came with it. One of the special ed programs took her under their wing did some testing and found she was qualified for special ed. During that special ed time, she was withdrawn and not really functioning right, but as they worked with her, she was capable of learning to be responsible for part of the coffee shop. It broke her shell and she was able to get up and talk about it.

The other day during our meeting, they brought this young lady in and she actually got up and talked. She stuttered at the first but then all of a sudden, it just came out. That is what jobs and working can do. It is not always about the academic part, especially in Indian Country.

If I could use this arm a little better, I would be able to explain because I too am like that, to express myself, to be able to show the point the importance of losing our child and what is happening today and the help we need. It needs to be equal on how it is shared and brought to us. Most important is the responsibility of growing up and being able to work and able to know that I have someplace to go.

Senator DAINES. Thank you for the great story, Councilman Clifford.

I am out of time. Thank you, Mr. Chairman.

The CHAIRMAN. Thank you, Senator Daines.

Senator Heitkamp?

Senator HEITKAMP. Thank you, Mr. Chairman.

I do not think anyone here thinks that suicide is anything other than a symptom of what are clearly conditions that many children on the reservation and in Indian Country exist in, creating stress. In the last Congress, we held a hearing on trauma-based interventions and had some amazing testimony relative to altered brain chemistry as a result of stress. I want to address some of this with you, Doctor.

At Johns Hopkins, an institution really close to Washington, the researchers think they have discovered a chemical alteration in a single human gene linked to stress reaction that if confirmed in larger studies could give doctors a blood test that may tell them who is at risk and who is not. They believe that this genetic mutation caused as a result of exposure to stress and trauma is a gene known as SKA–2. By looking at brain samples from people who had poor mental health and healthy people, the researchers found in that sample from people who had died by suicide, levels of SKA–2 that were significantly reduced.

You can go back to the work being done in Montana on stress and trauma relative to brain chemistry. I think a lot of what we always talk about is treating symptoms. We are going to do intervention, we are going to build resiliency, when this problem is a systemic-based problem driven by trauma and stress. I am not a doctor but I think when you look at these issues, I think you have to come to a clear understanding of what we are dealing with.

How can we integrate some of the new brain chemistry research that we are seeing now into the programs you are talking about? How can we do a better job modernizing the way we look at this?

As the Senator from Utah and I know, because we both served as Attorneys General, we were talking about this problem in the 1990s, we talked about this problem the last decade and we still are talking about this problem and guess what? It has not gotten any better. It has gotten worse.

What about a new idea and taking a new look at brain research and what we can do to fashion or model better intervention programs?

Dr. LaFromboise. That is a heavy one.

Basically, here are a few things I would think about. You are talking about basically determining whether a person has experienced this trauma. It is also the case with screening which people are very resistant to but by early screening, you would be able to know a lot about a person to begin with.

Having had a child who experienced language learning disabilities, when I was learning about that, I can remember one of the people doing the assessments saying after a certain point, it does not matter how it happened or the fact it is there, it is now what are you going to do. Yes, we do need to improve assessment and to be able to determine this, to know whether it is there or not.

Senator Heitkamp. I can tell you stories of children who have been involved in anti-suicide programs who have been model children who later committed suicide. Sometimes interventions are not adequate.

Dr. LaFromboise. Part of the intervention is also turning that around. In terms of even changing brain chemistry, the coping aspect of it, because what will you do once you get everyone diagnosed? There are still people who are functioning every day, carrying on with their lives, that need to keep going.

Some of my colleagues said actually the article, the last one cited on my testimony by Wexler, probably the best researchers that I know of in Native American suicide, are there and we struggle with this all the time.

Some people will say they think I am na?ve in terms of focusing on these interventions. They say we have to change the marginalization, the oppression and all these things. Yes, we do and we need to treat the people in the meantime.

It may take three generations, even if we change all these things. What do we do with all the people in the meantime that do need help and are even mildly exposed to trauma and can benefit from these activities?

Senator Heitkamp. I have just a little bit of time.

If we keep doing what we are doing right now and do everything the way we have done it and we are all here in ten years, do you think we have a better result?

Dr. LaFromboise. We are not doing enough right now. I am just highlighting the potential if we were using effective programs. We are not doing that now.

Senator Heitkamp. I think we need to modernize effective programs. I think there have been a number of examples, if I can take a minute, as we look at this and as we look at some of the tribal-based strategies treating trauma, identifying historic trauma, identifying some of the neurological issues that we have and being able to transition some of that new thinking into interventions, and when we look at this being done in places like the Menominee who have been able to double graduation rates. I just want to bring a broader kind of new development and new research into the discussion.

Thank you, Mr. Chairman.

The CHAIRMAN. Thank you very much, Senator Heitkamp. Senator Murkowski?

STATEMENT OF HON. LISA MURKOWSKI, U.S. SENATOR FROM ALASKA

Senator MURKOWSKI. Thank you, Mr. Chairman.

It is always interesting listening to my colleague from North Dakota because of the issues you raise. The Chairman and I were just talking about how many hearings on suicide in Indian Country we have had before this Committee. Again, we are not seeing the statistics get much better.

The one thing I have noted is that we are just kind of changing the deckchairs here. It used to be that Alaska was number one, now it is Montana and Wyoming tied for number one, New Mexico tied for number three and Alaska has dropped to number four.

We have not really solved the problems. We are still continuing the discussions. In the meantime, we are losing our children.

In addition, to follow up on your line of inquiry about the mental trauma and some of the research we are seeing, look at our increasing levels of suicide amongst our military, amongst our veterans, those who have experienced some level of trauma.

Again, I am with you. I am not the doctor here but it does lead you to conclude that maybe we need to be looking at some other areas. I would certainly be interested in working with my friend on this.

I look at where we seem to be having some limited success in my State. About four years ago now, we had a town hall on suicide in Bethel and brought out as many people who were willing to talk about suicide right after a horrible rash of suicide in some of the villages up north.

In fairness, it was much of the same conversation that we hear around here until we came to the very end where some of the children, the students I had invited from some of the villages that had been impacted, rose to speak.

It was painful listening to them because they stood in the center in front of all these grownups and elders and could not speak. They were so brave that they would not let themselves sit down. They stood for a minute in silence gathering the courage to speak about what had happened in their village. One young woman made the comment that yes, suicide was kind of a normal teenage thing. It ripped at your heart.

I think it was from that roundtable that we have seen within the White Cage Sea, they identified four different villages, Hooper Bay, Chevak, Scammon and Alakanuk who have had exceptionally high rates of suicide. They began to focus specifically on these communities.

In their message to me, since they have been doing that, they have experienced no suicides to this point in time. What are they doing? It is the culturally-based programs. It is gatherings, pot luck lunches, arts and crafts activities, making fish traps, and the talking circles.

Some of the other things that we look to, there is a gentleman from Tanana, Vernon Stickman, Sr., who lost a daughter to suicide in 2010. He walks the Yukon River during the wintertime, 140 miles from community to community to raise awareness.

Is that helping? I do not know. Is he as one person who does not have a program, who does not have a budget, just saying I am willing to do whatever it takes to get some attention to this, to shine some kind of a spotlight on it, to deal with my own personal grief, I think, as a dad.

I look to where we can be making a difference. I just met with some of our leaders in suicide education and prevention yesterday. I said, James, what is the one thing we could do that would make a difference. It is the mental health professionals.

It seems to me so much that particularly with youth suicide, it has to be the kids that are there for one another, saying I am there for you. As we talk about these programs, I hope that we are not just talking as adults in a room, talking about funding, budgets and what the MSPI program is doing to make progress.

I really hope that it is designed to involve the young people for their ideas. I think it was not until those young people spoke up in Bethel that we really started to talk about it. It was not until the young people at AFN two years up ago spoke up from Tanana and called out the parents, the adults, the elders and said, we are tired of being the victims of neglect, sexual assault, violence, and suicide. Wake up, grownups. What are you going to do about it? Anything that we can be doing that is bringing in our young people for the solutions, I think has to be key.

Mr. McSwain, I want to ask you one quick question regarding the MSPI program. We think it is making some progress. We are hearing from some of the groups in our State that it is. I have been a supporter of it. I think it is culturally relevant. I think it is getting us going in the right place.

I have been told on a few occasions that the overall structure and the management currently inhibit the program from being used to its full potential. I was told by a group in Alaska that some questions they have submitted to the program virtually went unanswered. I do not know much more beyond that.

I am wondering whether it is a lack of resources that is complicating effectively running this program or if you are aware of any other obstacles that we have faced with regard to the MSPI?

Mr. MCSWAIN. Senator, I believe that the MSPI program is doing some great things. I think it is one of those where it is at the community level and the community is directing it. In all of our programs, whether it is STPI or MSPI, when the community has its own design on what they want to do with the resources, they know how to move forward. That is what is making the progress in that program.

It has been six years since we have had it in place. We will be doing a full review of the six years to see what the successes are and what improvements ought to happen. We are doing that this year.

I liked your other comment about the kids. That struck a tone with me. The one area we have not done a real good job about and we are going to do that, is simply having kids get together, having our service units. I recommend to the tribes that they do it as well. The tribes are really interested.

We start talking about the pathways, hiring students as a GS–1, GS–2 or GS–3 and having them provide support to us. I think a comment was made by Dr. LaFromboise about the schools and the security they feel.

You can imagine what I felt when I was worried about suicides and the schools were letting out in the Northern Plains. What is going to happen to all those kids? Do they have any structure?

That is a part of it and certainly a conversation we are having with all of the MSPI recipients as to what they can do for kids. This expansion we have proposed for 2016 in Generation Indigenous is about kids. It is building on the MSPI.

If you are having questions, if there are concerns from folks from Alaska, ask us and we will look into it.

Senator MURKOWSKI. Thank you, Mr. Chairman.

The CHAIRMAN. Thank you, Senator Murkowski.

Senator Udall.

Senator UDALL. Thank you, Mr. Chairman.

Mr. McSwain, Senator Heitkamp asked about brain research in this area, new brain research and the discussion with Dr. LaFromboise. Do you have any thoughts on that from the Indian Health Service perspective or your work with SAMHSA? Is this a fruitful area? Is this something we should be looking into, some of those latest things being discovered?

Mr. McSWAIN. I do not think we can leave any rock unturned, the brain being one of them. I think our health care delivery system will be looking to other folks, the professionals, if you will, certainly the NIH folks and others that do this kind of work for anything that can help.

It is not going to be as easily magical as that. In my view, it is going to be a partnership that happens between the Administration and the tribes. That is the partnership that will be able to give them the tools.

Making an observation, some of our communities are just paralyzed because of the suicides. We have to do more to help them feel they can do something. That is part of our administrative responsibility.

In terms of science, I will leave that to scientists.

Senator UDALL. Thank you. Thank you for your work in this area.

Teresa, thank you for your work with the Zuni Pueblo. Longtime Pueblo in New Mexico really care about their young people. When they learn what is the right thing to do, they really invest in it. It is good to see that you were out there.

I am wondering, were they able to incorporate these things into the schools and other areas in order to make a real impact?

Dr. LAFROMBOISE. It has made a significant difference. I think Mr. Lewis testified here in 2008 that they had basically reversed the suicide rate and it is seldom happening now. It is a required course in the high school.

I was there a few years ago and actually the families were having meetings in the evening because they were doing more cultural adaptation of it.

Senator UDALL. What should a community do if they have one of these clusters? I have been to several in my tribal communities when in a period of weeks they lose two or three of their young people. They may not have had this happen before.

How do you view the steps that should be taken to tackle it if they run into that kind of situation?

Dr. LaFromboise. First of all, I have to defer to people who are clinical interventionists on the ground. I have focused in recent years more on prevention.

In essence, I think having a rapid response and bringing in people who have dealt with trauma and also communities is critical. I am sure that Chairman Seki knows more about that from their experience with the trauma that happened years ago at Red Lake.

Basically, there is work in place but there are better people to respond to that question.

Senator Udall. Chairman Seki, would you like to respond?

Mr. Seki. Are you talking about the trauma?

Dr. LaFromboise. The suicide clusters.

Senator Udall. Yes, the suicide clusters.

Mr. Seki. We suffered high suicide incidents and suicide ideation by our children for many years. The major factors underlying the suicide rates are long standing substance abuse, poverty and generation trauma. This is not a cluster but a sustained rise in suicide rates.

Having more counselors and meeting with the students individually is crucial. Right now the ratio is one counselor per 290 students. It does not work. We have to have more counselors and more social workers to address these issues we have in our school system and our reservations.

It is not easy to fix just like that. It takes time because people suffer a long, long time. When it happened in Red Lake, people are still suffering at this time. The suicides are happening on our reservation.

Some counselors I talk with say it happens. One happened in one area and then there are others, these are friends, saying they want to do it, more or less seven or more people doing it at the same time. It is work that needs to be corrected by adding more counselors and social workers working together.

Everything starts at home with parental involvement. Poverty and no jobs, create more jobs for the families so they can address these issues with their children because everything leads to drug and alcohol abuse when all this is not in place.

It is very hard for our people back in Red Lake, what we face, to continue trying to address these issues with our Native youth because it is a problem all over, not just at Red Lake. I heard Pine Ridge and this lady talking about different ideas and Mr. McSwain.

These are the things that you, as elected officials, have to come up with ways for us, tribal nations, to invest in tribes so they can fix their infrastructure, come up with ideas to improve the system and what is happening with our youth on our reservations.

We need help. It is not just us but everyone. Everyone has to be involved all the way from the parents. You have to listen, as Senator Murkowski said, to the children's ideas. You have to listen to the youth, what their ideas are. Pick that up and use that as working together to resolve these issues.

It is not going to happen if we keep cutting funds to the reservations because of sequestration. Those are the dollars they lose for creating more jobs, for bringing in more counselors and social service workers.

If sequestration is reversed, it could be fixed in six months or less if it goes back to 2013. That is not enough, there is more to it, to create these programs. We need more culturally based programs for our people to understand the culture and teach our youth what it is to be a Shanabe person because it is not easy. It is hard.

I am just now chairman for a year and I am very sensitive talking about our youth because I know they have problems. I like visiting with them, talking to them and finding ways to resolve their issues.

Also bullying is a concern but it leads right back to the parents. Parenting needs to be focused because it all starts at the home.

Senator UDALL. Mr. Chairman, you are absolutely right. I think you are right about the underlying causes. We have to tackle those. We have to invest the resources. We should not be cutting in terms of the kinds of resources that are there.

I thank this panel very much and yield back.

The CHAIRMAN. Thank you, Senator Udall.

Senator Franken.

Senator FRANKEN. Mr. Chairman, thank you, for what you just said.

When we are faced with the realities, you sort of wonder where to begin because whether you begin with unemployment, that is a big place to start. I have been to Pine Ridge which is I think 75 percent unemployment. What is the unemployment rate at Red Lake?

Mr. SEKI. About 50 percent.

Senator FRANKEN. We talk about trauma. I read a book called How Children Succeed, and it talked about adverse childhood experiences which lead to trauma. The author talks about extreme poverty, alcohol and drug abuse at home, abuse, whether it is neglect, physical abuse or sexual abuse, of you witnessing domestic abuse when you are a child, and living in a dangerous neighborhood where you see violence.

American Indians, on top of that, have seen cultural trauma for generations, so where do you begin? You witness the other families' domestic violence when you have poor housing and you see drug abuse too, even if your own parents are not using.

I went to a rehab facility in Bemidji, Oshki Manidoo, a White Earth facility. I visited the kids there. Every child I talked to had started using with their parents. We have very systemic problems here. Where do you start?

Mr. Chairman, I think you are right. You start with jobs but you also start with the funding that we do for programs. You are right. It was Buck Jourdain at the time, Buck I know longer than you and I apologize that during my introduction, I think I said Seki instead of Seki.

President Bush said, we won't forget you. During the last sequestration, there were less funds coming in for school counselors and during that time there were suicides. The very first thing we can do is fund these professionals.

Yes, these professionals engage the kids. These professionals should be professionals about engaging with children. We cannot depend on children to solve this themselves. We are the adults. We are supposed to be the adults. We are the grownups here. We are the Indian Affairs Committee.

We are supposed to fight for funding for you because which other of our colleagues will do that if not us. My challenge is to my colleagues on this Committee. We have these hearings in which we hear this testimony and our other colleagues in the Senate do not even hear this.

Our job on this Committee is to fight for you, to fight for your kids. We are supposed to be the grownups. We cannot put this off on the kids. Yes, a good counselor knows how to engage kids. A good counselor knows much better than we do how to get kids talking to other kids and kids involved in activities talking to other kids.

We have adult responsibilities here. One of our adult responsibilities is not to take away school counselors during sequestration and not sit here when the Director of the Bureau of Indian Affairs has to defend the budget and the numbers are woefully lacking and embarrassing.

I had questions about lots of things but it is our responsibility to be funding the things we know work and to fight for economic development in your communities, to fight for Indian energy, to fight for jobs but to also fight for the services that you need.

I apologize. I can only apologize for myself, that we have not been doing enough for your kids and for you.

Thank you, Mr. Chairman.

The CHAIRMAN. Thank you, Senator Franken.

Director McSwain, in briefings with the Committee staff and during a visit last week to Pine Ridge by one of our staff, it became clear that the agencies within the Department of Health and Human Services do not actually sufficiently coordinate with each other.

Regardless of the level of support available, there does not seem to be sufficient coordination with each other or with agencies and other departments like the Bureau of Indian Affairs, the Bureau of Indian Education, to the effect that there are devastating consequences.

What is your plan to fix this coordination and communication gap we heard about in last week's visit to Pine Ridge?

Mr. McSWAIN. I am not so certain I know what you heard from Pine Ridge. Certainly from all the calls I have been on leading up to it, the coordination has increased. In fact, the Office of Secretary has taken a lead role and given us all assignments. We are all reporting on those assignments as we move forward.

I think for the first time, as a department, we are all together. I know the department is reaching out to other people who have the ability to help like Education, DOI and so forth.

I have seen a marked increase on coordination, particularly the ones with whom we work closely like HRSA, SAMHSA and such. That coordination has really increased. We just have to make sure that it is always there for the next crisis.

The CHAIRMAN. I think it makes a point that it needs to always be there. In my discussions with Secretary Burwell last week, I got the impression from her that now the focus was there but you wish it had been for a long period of time. We want to make sure that focus continues, not just in one location, but throughout the communities. I am going to call on you to please continue that level of focus that is there right now but had not been and we cannot let it fall apart.

Mr. McSWAIN. Yes, and I would say Secretary Burwell took a very personal interest in this. She said, we have to fix this. She told us all to step up and step up together. She put the Deputy Secretary in charge of making sure we did that.

The CHAIRMAN. She mentioned that too.

Native suicide is not a new issue. We were dealing with this on the Wind River Reservation back on the 1980s. It is still not clear to me that the Administration is operating under an evidence-based plan to prevent suicide across Indian Country. That is not just this Administration. I think we have seen this now for decades.

Is there a plan in effect? If there is a plan in effect, it is obviously not working and needs to be reevaluated. As the head of the HIS, you are leading the effort. Your goal should be, of course, to bring the suicide rate for Native youth to zero. Task force meetings and planning sessions are not accomplishing that. When can we expect to see real results?

Mr. McSWAIN. We have something in the statement that talks about Zero Suicide which is really going to enable us to engage the system and be able to track certainly a lot better than the data we have had so far.

We actually have relied on our health IT system to tell us a lot, but we have to reach out beyond that to be able to know what is happening in the community as opposed to just what is happening in our clinics.

As you know, we have always said we are a health care provider, we do not get out in the community but we have to engage the community and be able to report that as well so we can have a complete data picture of what we are doing so we can have a baseline and be able to come back to you and say, these are the results. We have done that with the trends analysis but we need to do more.

The CHAIRMAN. Chairman Seki, in your testimony you outlined how Red Lake could end suicide at your reservation. Specifically, you highlighted expanding your wellness counselor program. The wellness counselors are social workers located in the schools and are critical frontline components of your suicide prevention plan.

Can you explain the advantages of having the counselors in the schools and how they have actually helped reduce suicides at Red Lake?

Mr. SEKI. As I stated before, counselors meet with students individually. They have times set aside to talk with the students that have problems, talking about suicides or domestic issues at home. They address these with them individually, giving them a plan on how to resolve this and continue working with them.

Having only two counselors at each school is not enough. They need more counselors so the counselors have fewer students to speak to regarding the issues happening with our youth.

It is very important that the agencies funding our youth counselors plus our social service people, that they continue to invest in them because we need more people, more of those counselors, more social workers to address these issues so that our students can go to someone when they have problems.

The wellness counselors and social workers address these and help them, help our youth.

The CHAIRMAN. Thank you.

Councilman Clifford, last week during the visit I mentioned one of our staff members made to Pine Ridge, they heard a lot about problems with the Rapid City Regional West and Indian Health Service facility.

Perhaps the most concerning was the impression among some community leaders that going to that facility did not really make a difference for Native youth. We heard that young people who are sent to the Regional West for being suicidal or attempting suicide often actually committed suicide later.

I wanted to get kind of a follow-up from you. Some have suggested that sexual abuse is a major driving factor of Native youth suicide. There was a long editorial and story in the New York Times about that specific part of it.

Based on your experience, could you talk a little bit about that, particularly as an educator who is at the front lines and helping young people every day? What role do you think sexual abuse and domestic abuse play with regard to the youth suicide question?

Mr. CLIFFORD. First of all, whenever you combat whatever issue it is, we have to be stirred up and bring the issue forward. What happens on the Pine Ridge Reservation locally has a lot to do with alcohol and drugs, overwhelmed with them.

Sexual abuse is amongst some of the crimes committed that are not dealt with. It is like getting a cut and it being able to fester and you are not taking care of it. Eventually, it is going to infect your whole body.

The same is true of a physical attack on your mind emotionally, that festers to the point of where there is hopelessness and it is there. The reality of it is that it is there. I am here to tell you that the hopelessness is there.

The lack of funding of different programs, I specifically worked in education for a great number of years and I am really glad you brought up funding disparities that go on. When we talk about counselors, guidance counselors versus a psychological counselor, there is a big difference there.

What use do I have for one of them counselors or both of them counselors? I have use for both of them. I have mentioned that in dealing with some of these things in our life and education, we seem to put an individual education plan forward to children identified with special needs.

In reality, I feel studying all these years, each and every young person from K to forever how long they go to school, having individual education plans set forth not just for the special needs children.

As we go through our life and place judgment on these children, I want to say judgment because that is how we use the data that is provided, they are gains, they are individual growth gains, not a standard that says all third graders are like that, not all seventh graders are like that but an individual education plan that would monitor that child and young person's self, not rated amongst each other.

The sexual abuse that does go on does happen on the Pine Ridge Indian Reservation and it relates to the poverty.

I would like to quickly mention the disparity on some funding. We are underfunded in all schools nationwide, Indian education, operation and maintenance, and transportation. We take the ISEP dollars designed for children to learn and the title dollars and we use them to fix our schools. We are using them to pay our light bill and to pay for propane to keep them warm.

I can go on forever on that. In the case of that, there needs to be money there. All of this work is critical.

I would like to ask that the Committee support our efforts to save the lives of our children. We need long term solutions, not a quick band-aid today.

Thank you.

The CHAIRMAN. Thank you very much, Councilman Clifford.

Do any of you have a short closing comment on the things you have heard said today? We are in the middle of roll call votes. I think we have a number of them now and the roll call vote has already been called so we have to summarize.

Director McSwain, any last thoughts?

Mr. McSWAIN. I think this will require us, as the Administration, to work very, very closely with the communities and engage the communities where they are engaged on the issues. They need the tools and we need to provide the tools to be able to address this particular issue.

Right now we are finding that many of our communities are, as I mentioned earlier, rather paralyzed. There is something they want to do. In fact, my weekly calls with President Steele to be able to see how he is doing and how the tribe is doing, as an Administration, we have to do more of that.

The CHAIRMAN. Mr. Clifford?

Mr. CLIFFORD. I would recommend the following: providing emergency funding for substance abuse and suicide prevention and mental health care; commit to economic development and infrastructure on the Pine Ridge. I ask respectfully to remove the jurisdictional restrictions and fund tribal police and courts and focus on education for our youth suicide epidemic. It would probably be best fought in the schools.

Lastly, acknowledge the government's treaty obligation to fully fund all these programs.

Thank you.

The CHAIRMAN. Mr. Seki?

Mr. SEKI. Thank you for giving us this opportunity. I want to thank the panel here that spoke regarding the suicides.

The thing I will keep addressing is the sequestration, to stop it, to put back the funds for the tribes so they can address these suicides happening on our reservations. Pine Ridge alluded to grants.

That is not the solution. Long term funding like SAMHSA and DOG is the solution. Put them through the 638 agreements, not short term because short term does not work. They only last as long as the grant and then it is over. Then we are back to square one again.

I ask you as the Committee to invest in tribal nations for infrastructure, for economic development, for tribes to create jobs for our safety and for our generations to come, our youth.

Thank you.

The CHAIRMAN. Thank you, Mr. Seki.

Dr. LaFromboise?

Dr. LAFROMBOISE. In addition to all that has been said, I think we need to remember it is very important to strengthen the workforce of American Native and Alaska Natives in the fields of mental health. We need to look at funding beyond psychiatry and psychology with the Indian Health Service to include social work and Masters level people. They can work in collaboration with the schools to deliver some of these programs. There are programs proven to be effective. They just need the staffing with which to do that.

I also realize that I pushed the issue of evidence-based but do agree with what has been said today, that there are many practices the community knows work. Unfortunately, because they have not been proven through scientific methods, they often are looked upon as less than and they are not. They are equal to, if not more powerful. We just do not have the resources for those to continue as much as they should in full force.

I want to be on record as having said, there is really a balance between traditional practices and then some of these other more western-based practices that we have proven that do work with Native kids.

The CHAIRMAN. Thank you.

I appreciate your comments. There may be some written questions by other members of the Committee who were unable to be here with us today. The hearing record will be open for two weeks.

I am going to remind the Administration that our work is not complete. I look forward to continued dialogue, including Committee briefings, listening sessions, and hearings in the weeks to come.

I want to thank all the witnesses for your time and testimony.

The hearing is adjourned.

[Whereupon, at 4:12 p.m., the Committee was adjourned.]